Intensive
Caring

"*Intensive Caring* is an essential Catholic guide for serious illness and end-of-life care. Dr. Natalie King's sincere compassion and respect for the human person make this weighty subject wonderfully approachable. Using practical clinical experience and extensive knowledge of the Catholic Church's teachings, King delivers sound guidance for those making difficult medical decisions for themselves or a loved one."

Michelle K. Stanford, MD
President of the Catholic Medical Association

"Dr. King draws wisdom from her palliative care experience and navigates the complex ethical and theological terrain surrounding suffering and the dying process with compassion and great skill. This practical guide is a must-read for Catholics facing serious illness and their caregivers, as well as an indispensable guide for clinicians, chaplains, and pastors."

Michael Garrido, MAPS
Vice President of Mission Integration
Emory St. Joseph's Hospital

"As a contemplative, a caregiver, and a cancer patient, I found Dr. King's tremendous resource, *Intensive Caring*, to be the most helpful book I've read on end-of-life issues. King's expertise in palliative care shines through compassionately in this comprehensive and clear guide to everything from medical procedures, choices, and how to make decisions to the Church's teachings on medical ethics and the dignity of the human person. A terrific companion for Catholics contemplating the challenges surrounding death and dying, this is also a beautiful manual for living life to its fullest with faith and trust in the goodness of God's love for each of us. This will be my new go-to book for anyone facing a challenging diagnosis!"

Lisa M. Hendey
Author of *The Grace of Yes*

"As a caregiver, I longed for the information that is contained in this book! Faithful people want to do what is right for the sick. But what is right? And whom do we call on to support us and our loved ones when facing serious illness? I have heard Dr. King speak about her work with great love and deep compassion. Her compassion spills out of this book, giving important guidance to and about the seriously ill."

Rev. Richard Doerr
Pastor of Our Lady of Mt. Carmel Church
Carmel, Indiana

NATALIE KING, MD

Intensive Caring

A PRACTICAL HANDBOOK FOR CATHOLICS ABOUT SERIOUS ILLNESS AND END-OF-LIFE CARE

AVE MARIA PRESS AVE Notre Dame, Indiana

Nihil Obstat: Reverend Monsignor Michael Heintz, PhD
   Censor Librorum

Imprimatur: Most Reverend Kevin C. Rhoades
   Bishop of Fort Wayne–South Bend
   Given at Fort Wayne, Indiana, on 15 May, 2024

The *Nihil Obstat* and *Imprimatur* are official declarations that a book or pamphlet is free of doctrinal or moral error. No implication is contained therein that those who have granted the *Nihil Obstat* or *Imprimatur* agree with its contents, opinions, or statements expressed.

Founded in 1865, Ave Maria Press is a ministry of the United States Province of Holy Cross.

www.avemariapress.com

Paperback: ISBN-13 978-1-64680-318-7

E-book: ISBN-13 978-1-64680-319-4

Cover image © Simon Lee/Unsplash.

Cover design by Andy Wagoner.

Text design by Esther Moody.

Printed and bound in the United States of America.

Library of Congress Cataloging-in-Publication Data is available.

This book is dedicated to the patients I have cared for and their families. You have been some of my greatest teachers in the strength you exhibit despite suffering and limitations, in the devotion you demonstrate in caring for each other, and in the courage you exemplify as you face difficulties. It has been such a privilege to care for you and to witness such great beauty and love.

CONTENTS

ACKNOWLEDGMENTS

Intensive Caring has been a true labor of love and the result of such an unexpected yet rich and beautiful journey in my life. I give glory to God for the talents, opportunities, and gifts he has bestowed upon me and pray my life and ministry can bring honor to him.

To the spiritual directors and professional mentors who have aided in my formation along the way. You have made an indelible mark on my life.

To the friend who opened the door for me to Ave Maria Press, and for all at Ave who have helped support this book, particularly my editor. It has been a lovely experience working with you.

To those in the Catholic medical community who shared their time and professional expertise in reviewing this manuscript. I am so grateful to be in the trenches with you.

To the many friends and relatives who have provided prayers and emotional support as I work to follow God's call in my life professionally and personally. Thank you for knowing and loving me.

To my mother: you have always enthusiastically supported my work and believed in my call to help people in this unique way. Thank you for the gift of my life, for your tireless ability to listen to my heart, and for all your love.

To my daughter: the timing of your entrance onto the scene provided a beautiful opportunity for me to put this project together. From being in the womb during the writing of the manuscript, to being in the world during the editing, you have been with me. I pray that you may, too, in your life have opportunities to let your passions flourish and give glory to God.

To my beloved husband: thank you for your unwavering support and encouragement of my ministry, for helping me bring to life the inspirations from my prayers, for being a model of virtuous living, and for loving me and willing my good.

I SEE YOUR STRESS AND WANT TO HELP

Often, when someone learns that I am a physician, they ask what my specialty is. When I share that I am a palliative medicine physician, they usually look at me quizzically. I then explain that I care for people with serious illness or, sometimes, nearing the end of life. If the conversation does not just end rather awkwardly right then, I typically get one of these three responses:

> "That is so sad! How are you not depressed all the time?"

> "Oof! It takes a really special person to do that kind of work."

> "Wow, that is really beautiful! Tell me more about what you do."

Which response I get tends to correlate with where the person is in their own understanding and acceptance of mortality. As much as I would like to say I frequently get the third response, it is in fact the least common. Our culture just does not help us feel comfortable with sickness, suffering, and death. We tend to think and talk about these things as simply bad, rather than as stages of life, which, though difficult—sometimes terribly so—are nonetheless experiences over which we humans can exercise more control than we are sometimes able to see or understand.

Many of us have never had helpful examples to follow of individuals and families navigating medical decisions toward the goal of a peaceful death. We are not regularly introduced to important skills that can help us think and talk about human suffering, debility, and death, let alone make important healthcare decisions based on our deeply held convictions and values. Consequently, many people simply sidestep decisions until they are forced to deal directly and personally with them.

For Catholics this can feel particularly stressful, as we desire to follow what the Church teaches, but the teachings can often appear confusing in themselves and perplexing in how to appropriately apply them. Catholic belief contradicts growing cultural perceptions of suffering and dying as nothing more than a stage of life to be tolerated (or expedited) until we die. Our faith teaches that there is so much more involved here. Even in the process of dying, we have immense dignity, and there are continued opportunities for meaning, growth, and the ability to love and be loved.

As a fellow Catholic and a palliative medicine physician, I see and hear your stress, and I wrote this book to help you be as well prepared as you can be when you and those you love come up against end-of-life choices regarding medical care and well-being. I wrote for you who are undertaking advance care planning and you who find yourselves in more urgent situations—when tough choices need to be made in the very near future. I wrote to equip and empower you, as others have empowered me all along my faith journey, which seems to deepen in tandem with my work in medicine.

I was raised Catholic and attended Catholic schools through my undergraduate education. And it was in college that my faith really took root and grew significantly deeper. I will be forever grateful to a spiritual director I had at the University of Notre Dame who told me that in addition to my calling to marriage and family life, I likely had a professional vocation to medicine. Although I do not recall a specific moment when this career path became clear as the right one for me, when I look back, I'm sure that my childhood experiences were highly influential.

When I was eight, my beloved grandmother had a massive stroke and transitioned to living in a nursing care facility on the third floor of the community hospital near our town of Jeffersonville, Indiana. The stroke left Mawmaw minimally verbal, incontinent, bed- and wheelchair-bound, and with a feeding tube for nutrition. My vibrant and active grandmother, previously with a job at a local department store and with a great talent for crocheting, was unalterably changed. She lived like that for three years before she died. My family visited her often, and I remember reading a Laura Ingalls Wilder book to her and playing piano for her and other residents. My father and his six siblings signed up on a calendar in her room for the days they would visit so not a day would pass when Mawmaw did not have someone coming by. My grandfather, Mawmaw's husband of fifty-two years, had previously suffered a stroke and was no longer able to drive, so he would take the public bus to visit Mawmaw each day. He was not a verbose gentleman, but he would spend his days with his beloved bride, simply sitting next to her and holding her hand.

For nearly as long as I can remember, my father had a myriad of health issues, including a bout with colon cancer when I was eleven. I also experienced the deaths of multiple elderly relatives. I felt deeply the loss of my last grandparent when I was just eleven years. I felt robbed of the special relationships between grandchild and grandparents and envied friends at school, particularly on grandparents' day.

In my teens I experienced death in an entirely different way through the trauma of losing two young people I knew quite well in dreadful car crashes. I am sure that all these intimate experiences of death and dying had a significant effect on me. Witnessing the strength that simple, honest acts of love and courage bring during the really hard things of life formed my understanding of dying and death as yet another part of one's journey through this earthly life. I learned early that while frightening, painful, and terribly disorienting, the end of life—faced with trust in God and in the company of loved ones—need not be. And in ways I do not yet entirely understand, these experiences predisposed me toward the work I now do. It seems absolutely clear to me that God was working in all of it.

When I reached medical school, I realized that I was not good at defending Catholic teachings and there were many things about Catholicism I did not fully understand. It also became clear early on that some things being taught in the classroom were antagonistic to Church teachings. Medical technology had paved the ways for groundbreaking things like embryonic stem cell research and cloning. Abortion, sterilization, and contraception were presented as commonplace and considered standard options for medical care. I felt pressure to involve myself and to bend and change my beliefs. It became very discouraging and unsettling, leading me to honestly ask myself, Would it be possible to integrate my faith into my medical practice? Could I successfully (and feasibly) in today's world be a physician and simultaneously adherent to my Catholic faith? I knew I could not just be Catholic on Sundays when I went to Mass and act differently the rest of the week. I was profoundly aware that patients would be coming to me vulnerable and seeking my expertise and guidance. Their bodies (and souls) would be in my hands. In a real, direct way, my soul would be on the line for the care I would provide and would not provide. I would have direct influence over the lives of others and would have to account for this at the end of my life. The gravity of all this was terrifying.

Providentially, I was put in contact with a wonderful priest and also some very supportive Catholic physicians who assured me I could be both a faithful Catholic and a successful medical doctor, even in today's world. I learned of good supportive resources and organizations to help me and met several other friends who encouraged and strengthened me on this journey. Catholic teachings on the sanctity of life, care of the vulnerable, and charity toward others particularly influenced me as I progressed in my medical training. I strove to serve God in the details of my patient care and tried to practice virtuous medicine in sanctifying my daily work. As I gained more experience and responsibilities, I grew in my ability to advocate for justice, stand up against injustice, and be unafraid to speak out when needed.

Graduating medical school, I planned to become an oncologist, a cancer doctor. Like most of my peers, I was there to learn how to diagnose, successfully treat, and ultimately heal patients from disease. So it was quite a dramatic change of perspective when I decided instead to specialize in caring for patients who usually cannot be cured or "fixed." Instead of working for a cure, my aim would be to creatively reduce suffering so that my patients could live the best lives possible for as long as possible. I believed this to be quite a worthy objective, a challenge, and a gift that I now continue to pursue.

I really enjoyed taking care of patients (and their families) in the intensive care unit, and I had a soft spot for geriatric patients. I owe much to a cardiologist on staff where I completed my internal medicine residency training, who noticed that I seemed distinctively comfortable communicating difficult news to patients and encouraged me to look into palliative care. Since there was no fellowship program for training in palliative care where I was, after some soul-searching and research, I took a leap and moved twelve hours away to a different state and completed one year of additional medical training. That was absolutely the right choice for me, and I came to realize the meaningful difference I could make by working creatively to help relieve the suffering and stress of patients—and their loved ones—who were going through serious illness and perhaps facing death.

After nearly a decade, I remain very passionate about this work, helping accompany people going through a serious illness to live the best life possible for as long as possible. It is such a privilege to get to know people beyond their disease, understand their values, and help them fulfill their healthcare goals—and many times their life goals—despite a difficult diagnosis.

During my first years of practice, I began receiving invitations to give educational presentations, primarily to Catholic audiences, on palliative medicine, hospice, and common end-of-life issues. The questions I repeatedly received at these talks demonstrated that many misunderstandings exist and these impart fear, making this time of life particularly stressful and frightening to navigate. My heart continues to break open and connect with the many people I meet in my audiences. I see patients who struggle with these tough medical issues and who want desperately to remain faithful to the Catholic faith they love. Addressing their questions and commitments became the foundation for this book.

This book contains ten chapters, each divided into common and crucial questions and answers regarding medical care options in serious illness and at the end of life. I debunk some of the myths that circulate around end-of-life care and review Catholic Church teaching throughout. It is written in a way that you can choose to read it straight through or select particular topics to focus on that are particularly applicable to your situation. I have incorporated patient examples and instructive stories from my own life to help you see connections and better apply your faith commitments to your own healthcare choices. I want to impart clarity and provide reassurance. The patients described in these chapters are based on real patients. Names and details have been altered to maintain anonymity.

In the conclusion of the book, I offer my own convictions about what makes for a happy death and the role that we Catholics can play to help our culture elevate the sanctity of life and safeguard the dignity of each human being from conception through natural death. Our Church provides us a rich tradition in these matters, offering us both practical and spiritual guidance. I also share some spiritual lessons and encouragement I have picked up along my life's journey. My hope and prayer are that these pages become for you a trusted, practical tool for tackling with confidence some of life's toughest decisions.

Lastly, there is an appendix at the end of the book with helpful resources, should you want to dig deeper into certain topics, as well as descriptions of related Church documents, if you desire to read more.

Thank you for having the interest and taking the time to read this book. I realize you may very well be in the midst of one of the most difficult health situations of your life or that of a loved one. May God bless you and grant you peace.

Chapter 1

MEDICAL CARE IN SERIOUS ILLNESS AND AT THE END OF LIFE

In this chapter, we will consider the general progression of serious illness and end-of-life medical issues. We'll examine what suffering related to illness can look like, and I will share a multifaceted approach to assessing how suffering is understood and confronted in contemporary Western culture. I will provide a general overview of what guidance Catholic teaching and tradition offers us as we contemplate how we want to live in illness, in suffering, and as we or our loved ones near the end of life on this earth.

MEET MR. W

Mr. W is an eighty-four-year-old gentleman with no living relatives. He has been diagnosed with Parkinson's disease, which is a chronic (incurable) and progressive (worsens over time) neurological condition. Through his disease course he has developed arthritis and problems with walking, and he therefore suffers occasional falls (one of which caused him to fracture his hip). He has begun to have difficulty swallowing and is having problems with aspiration, so that food or drink "goes down the wrong pipe." He is losing weight and the ability to speak. He has had several hospital admissions over the last year, many due to aspiration-related pneumonias.

WHEN IS IT APPROPRIATE TO BEGIN THINKING ABOUT END-OF-LIFE ISSUES RELATED TO MY OWN HEALTH SITUATION?

You may know someone like Mr. W. You may even be experiencing serious health limitations yourself. The fact that you have picked up this book and read this far means that you recognize the gravity of these sorts of issues and the importance of addressing them. (I thank you for this!) My hope is that as you continue reading, your questions will be answered, and you will be able to think through the issues and move toward greater clarity about how you would want your care and your life to look. I also hope this book will teach you how you can best advocate for loved ones. My aim is to provide information through the lens of what is realistic in medicine and also what the Catholic Church believes and teaches, so that you become better equipped to make an honest assessment for yourself.

If you are a healthy person, thinking about your life in the setting of serious illness or nearing the end of life may seem like a waste of time. You might be saying to yourself, "I do not have medical problems. I don't need to think about these things." You might even say, "I know that these things are important for people to think about, but I don't need to think about them right now and can put them off for a while." As a healthy person myself, I can understand where you are coming from. Who wants to spend time thinking about what their life may look like and how they would feel if they had a serious illness or were nearing the end of their life? It is not fun; it can seem downright depressing. Yet, as a physician who specializes in caring for people who have significant health issues and a limited life expectancy, I can tell you with honesty: it is never too early to begin thinking about these things.

As cliché and horrible as it may seem to think it, every time we get in the car we never know if it will be our last ride. We know we are finite beings and that at some point we will face our mortality, but we also operate under the assumption that this point is some far-off place in the future. But what if it is right around the corner?

How you feel about potential healthcare options and what you would want if you found yourself in a particular situation may be different than what you (or others) would expect. As unenjoyable as this exercise may seem, it is very important, and what you communicate about how you feel is a true gift for yourself, and for your loved ones.

When serious illness or a health crisis happens, few people are prepared. Never would they have considered a scenario in which they would be faced with big medical choices: Do I go on the ventilator? Do I go on dialysis? Do I get that major surgery? Unfortunately, in many of these scenarios the patient is not even able to choose for themselves because they are too sick to clearly understand and process the options to make the choice. So the people around them must make the decision for them.

Even having basic conversations with your loved ones about your thoughts and preferences regarding healthcare choices can give them meaningful information that will enable them to have peace that they are honoring your wishes and respecting your preferences (and documenting these is even better, as we will see in chapter 5). I recall countless times a family member hearkened back to "when Dad said he never wanted to be on machines" or "when Mom hated visiting Aunt Roberta in the nursing home and always said she could not live in a place like that." This little bit of information can go a long way in providing peace when we are in the midst of grief-stricken and traumatic situations.

How serious illness presents and takes a course is different for each person and varies according to their medical situation. Some of the most jarring situations can occur when someone gets in an accident, experiences some sort of trauma, or develops a bad infection that is life threatening. Suddenly, the person's life is seriously changed. In a situation such as cardiac arrest, someone often goes from highly functioning to nearly dead in minutes. Some diseases, such as cancer, can come up quite unexpectedly. A person may still be able to function quite normally despite having advanced disease and receiving aggressive treatments. And then suddenly, the person may be doing much worse and may be told they are nearing the end of life. Other illnesses, such as dementia or frailty often seen in elderly people, are typically characterized by a more gradual decline in function that at times may occur over years. And then there are other situations, such as chronic organ failure (caused by kidney, heart, or lung disease), where there are episodic times of decline and stabilization, which may happen over decades. Regardless of the trajectory, the decline that illness brings can be extremely difficult.

COURSE OF ILLNESS AND DECLINE

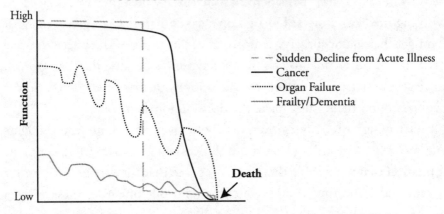

WHAT MIGHT SUFFERING LOOK LIKE IN THE WORLD TODAY?

We can all think back to situations in life where we have suffered. Be it a difficult pregnancy and childbirth, a painful injury, the discouraged longing of unanswered prayer, the loss of a loved one, or a financial crisis, suffering is ubiquitous to the human condition. Suffering related to serious illness can turn one's life upside down. Suffering is one of the toughest concepts to think about when you are considering the end-of-life period. Suffering is innately unattractive, and it is natural to want to avoid it. It is truly difficult to understand its purpose. The question of why a good God would allow suffering has always challenged humanity and continues to be a primary reason why people struggle with believing in God.[2]

Most people struggle with how to respond to suffering. It is something that makes most of us downright uncomfortable to think about, to witness, and to personally experience. It is a complex and many-layered reality. Having cared for many patients at their bedsides, I want to share with you what I believe are some social and cultural aspects of suffering that contribute to our experience of it, and to how we process and treat suffering today.

You will see how the secular world's and Catholic Church's approaches to suffering are quite at odds.

Technological Advances in Healthcare

Medical advances today have been amazing but also challenge the way medical care fits into one's life. We are now able to live longer, but often life includes chronic illnesses that require frequent and sometimes difficult interventions and hospitalizations (and rehospitalizations). Life-supportive advances like ventilators and dialysis machines are often able to ward off death much longer than before. But just because we *can*, does that always mean we *should*? The end-of-life period of one's life is becoming more difficult to define and predict and is lasting longer.

People are thus living longer with functional limitations or debility. This is particularly challenging in a culture that places high value on independence and autonomy (patient self-determination). I think much of what people refer to as "quality of life" comes from their understanding of physical health and functional ability to "do" things. When people become weaker, bedbound, demented, or get advanced organ failure and need things like dialysis, supplemental oxygen, or chronic blood transfusions, they may feel that the burden of suffering in their life impacts its value. Symptoms like chronic pain and debilitating shortness of breath can make previously simple activities become major obstacles.

Denial of Mortality

In general, our world today just does not like to think about death. And the healthcare system struggles to accept that death is a part of the human condition. Physicians fight so hard against a person's disease that at times the person who has the disease is almost forgotten. And if the disease "wins," and the person's body is succumbing to it despite the hard fight, it can feel like a personal loss for the physician. This unrealistic mindset is unfortunately bound for failure. Because at some point, the disease will win. And if not that disease, then a different one. Yet modern healthcare too often fails patients by not having the necessary conversations when ailments prove incurable or refractory to treatment options.

In a death-avoidant culture, it naturally follows, then, that any suffering associated with death should be avoided at all costs. If suffering cannot be avoided, a patient may wish to accelerate the process. Rather than proceed along the natural course of an incurable illness, a patient may feel pressure to bypass any potential suffering and plan the dying process on one's own terms. The desire for control here is a big factor. It is natural to wish for control of one's bodily functions and to not be dependent upon others (thinking, oftentimes incorrectly, that they are a "burden"). Some people would rather end their life on their own terms, even prematurely, to the point of avoidance of all physical decline or loss of control. And with increasing rates of social isolation and rampant loneliness in the culture, many who are facing the common fears inherent to a serious illness do not know where else to turn.

Misguided Compassion

The fears of personal suffering or of witnessing another person's suffering lead to modern society's growing sense of misguided compassion. It is hard to walk with someone in their suffering. Some might feel that it is merciful to hasten someone's death, to get rid of the suffering to the extent of killing the person. As section 4 of the Vatican's document on terminal illness and suffering, *Samaritanus Bonus*, states, "In the face of seemingly 'unbearable' suffering . . . so-called 'compassionate' euthanasia holds that it is better to die than to suffer, and that it would be compassionate to help a patient to die by means of euthanasia or assisted suicide. In reality, human compassion consists not in causing death, but in embracing the sick, in supporting them in their difficulties, in offering them affection, attention, and the means to alleviate the suffering." Compassion is not helping someone kill themselves. Yet you see this misguided compassion evident even in the name of the organization Compassion and Choices, an organization that works to advance physician-assisted suicide legislation across the United States.

Values in the "Throw-Away" Culture

There are increasing pressures about healthcare resources and financial costs, which is even more so exacerbated with the aging population. There is pressure to have an allocation of resources, with judgments on one's "quality of life," the utility of a person's life, and who deserves something and who does not.

Reflecting upon the current state of society, *Samaritanus Bonus* states: "Pope Francis has spoken of a 'throw-away culture' where the victims are the weakest human beings, who are likely to be 'discarded' when the system aims for efficiency" and high functioning "at all costs." He writes, "The current socio-cultural context is gradually eroding the awareness of what makes human life precious. In fact, it is increasingly valued on the basis of its efficiency and utility, to the point of considering as 'discarded lives' or 'unworthy lives' those who do not meet this criterion" (sec. 4).

Samaritanus Bonus goes on to discuss that when the culture speaks of one's "quality of life," it is referring to a "utilitarian anthropological perspective" that sees people

> in terms "primarily related to economic means, to 'well-being,' to the beauty and enjoyment of physical life, forgetting the other, more profound, interpersonal, spiritual and religious dimensions of existence." In this perspective, life is viewed as worthwhile only if it has, in the judgment of the individual or of third parties, an acceptable degree of quality as measured by the possession or lack of particular psychological or physical functions, or sometimes simply by the presence of psychological discomfort. According to this view, a life whose quality seems poor does not deserve to continue. Human life is thus no longer recognized as a value in itself. (sec. 4)

Western culture's emphasis on individualism views the other as a limitation or a threat to one's freedom, a "burden." What results is isolation and less dependence upon others, which is inherently disordered as at our deepest level we depend on God (and other people). With the culture's pre-rogative of radical autonomy, one has rights to do whatever one chooses. This thinking extends to whether or not to continue living (which is where concepts like physician-assisted suicide and euthanasia come in).

"This cultural phenomenon, which is deeply contrary to solidarity, John Paul II described as a 'culture of death' that gives rise to real 'structures of sin'" (sec. 4), and physician-assisted suicide and euthanasia arise as errone-ous solutions to the challenges of caring for terminal patients. The secular emphasis on freedom as the right to do whatever we desire to do is in direct opposition to the Christian concept of freedom: "To end the life of a sick person who requests euthanasia is by no means to acknowledge and respect their autonomy, but on the contrary to disavow the value of both their freedom, now under the sway of suffering and illness, and of their life by excluding any further possibility of human relationship, of sensing the meaning of their existence, or of growth in the theological life" (sec. 3).

While secular culture values one's "quality" of life and functional abilities, radical individualism, and avoidance of suffering in the name of compas-sion, Catholic belief emphasizes the inviolable sanctity of life, accompa-niment of the infirmed, and the viewing of others as gift. The Catholic Church teaches that one's life does not stop with a diagnosis and that one does not have less value now that there may be limitations—as Catholics, we believe that the value of life is so much more than that. People are meant to accompany others on the journeys that God directs—one's life is not one for them or others to personally direct. One's life is for one to give, not for one to take. Willfully ending one's life destroys the priceless creation they are and takes away autonomy and freedom rather than im-parting it.

Let us briefly look at the patient we met at the beginning of this chapter, Mr. W. Recall that he has been experiencing many health limitations and functional decline from Parkinson's disease. He is no longer able to be as independent. Perhaps he is considering a feeding tube given his swallowing difficulties or pondering whether or not he would want to go on a ventila-tor machine if he got a bad pneumonia. Has anyone on his medical team talked to him about his diagnosis and prognosis? Has he made any preparations as to his future decisions regarding his healthcare or his financial future? Has he communicated any of this to loved ones?

You can see through sharing Mr. W's story that serious illness can quickly lead to complex medical situations, with challenging decisions to be made. The suffering that patients experience is often multifaceted and unique to their individual situations. Navigating this can be quite daunting and is rarely "black and white." I will next highlight related Catholic teachings that help provide some additional guidance in this area.

WHAT DOES THE CATHOLIC CHURCH SAY IN GENERAL ABOUT THE END OF LIFE?

As Catholics, we accept that death is a part of life, and we do not believe that human life is absolute. We pray for respect for life "from conception to natural death." Life is not something that must be preserved at all costs, but we are called to protect and defend it. We see dignity in all human life, value the frail, disabled, and ill, and accompany the sufferer. We see our crucified Christ as the model for how to make suffering redemptive.

There are several Church documents that shed light on Catholic teachings and beliefs concerning the end of life (please see the appendix at the end of the book for further information). I will highlight a few here. To start with, the *Catechism of the Catholic Church* exhorts us to follow the Ten Commandments, the fifth of which forbids killing and teaches that human life is sacred as a creative act of God. Throughout Church teaching, there is an emphasis on life's inherent dignity. "Those whose lives are diminished or weakened deserve special respect. Sick or handicapped persons should be helped to lead lives as normal as possible" (*Catechism*, 2276). The dying should be cared for with respect and peace.

Two documents that St. John Paul II wrote that highlight issues relating to the end of life include the encyclical *Evangelium Vitae* (The Gospel of Life), published in 1995, and the apostolic letter *Salvifici Doloris* (On the Christian Meaning of Human Suffering), published in 1984. *Evangelium Vitae* describes the "incomparable worth of the human person" and details common threats to life in today's world, such as abortion, contraception, sterilization, research on embryos, and euthanasia. It articulates the Church's stance that human life is sacred and that humans are made for eternal life. John Paul II emphasizes how the goodness of God must be trusted, particularly in moments of physical affliction and suffering. "Man is not the master of life, nor is he the master of death. In life and in death, he has to entrust himself completely to the 'good pleasure of the Most High,' to his loving plan" (46).

Salvifici Doloris further explores the meaning and mystery of suffering. "Suffering seems to belong to man's transcendence: it is one of those points in which man is in a certain sense 'destined' to go beyond himself, and he is called to this in a mysterious way" (2). John Paul II then reviews how the experience of suffering is pervasive in the Bible, culminating in Christ's suffering on the Cross. As Christians, there is an invitation to share in Christ's suffering, an opportunity to participate in the Paschal Mystery of the Cross and Resurrection. All the weaknesses of our suffering "are capable of being infused with the same power of God manifested in Christ's Cross" (23). In suffering, you are making yourself especially open to the saving power of God, offered to us through Christ. In Christ "God has confirmed his desire to act especially through suffering, which is man's weakness and emptying of self, and He wishes to make His power known precisely in this weakness and emptying of self" (23). Therefore, suffering has great meaning and spiritual significance in our lives.

As introduced in the preceding section, the letter *Samaritanus Bonus* provides much relevant and practical information around Church teachings on the end of life. The Dicastery for the Doctrine of the Faith came out with the letter in 2020; its full title is *Samaritanus Bonus (The Good Samaritan): On the Care of Persons in the Critical and Terminal Phases of Life*. This document highlights current issues that are affronts to human dignity at its end—things like physician-assisted suicide and euthanasia.

This letter is for all who come into contact with the sick and dying: physicians, nurses, other healthcare workers, family members, priests, and other pastoral workers. It provides spiritual and practical guidance about the art of accompanying the sick and dying, following the model of the Good Samaritan, and speaks about the good of the field of palliative care.

"To those who care for the sick, the scene of the Cross provides a way of understanding that even when it seems that there is nothing more to do there remains much to do, because 'remaining' by the side of the sick is a sign of love and of the hope that it contains" (sec. 2).

As I shared in the preceding section, this document describes the culture of life that we need to aim for to combat the rampant "culture of death." It describes a culture of real accompaniment of the sick and dying, of practicing a *"contemplative gaze"* that views one's own life and that of others with "unique and unrepeatable wonder, received and welcomed as a gift." Having a contemplative gaze, one does not try to grasp at or take control of life, but welcomes it with its troubles and sufferings, and "guided by faith, finds in illness the readiness to abandon oneself to the Lord of life who is manifest therein" (sec. 1). Emulating the model of the Good Samaritan, we are called to take responsibility for others, caring for them in a way reflecting God's unconditional love, which gives life its true meaning.

And so we return again to our long-suffering patient Mr. W, who may well be nearing the end of his life. While secular culture may consider his quality of life poor and consider him a burden, looking at his care through a Catholic lens, we would focus on caring for him as a person with intrinsic value and dignity that is not lessened in the least by his infirmity and limitations. We would advocate for Mr. W to be cared for as lovingly as possible, with attention to his comfort and symptom management, and we would commit to helping him live the best life he can, working to educate him about his disease and prognosis, soliciting his opinion about his preferences regarding his care, and setting out to respect those preferences. We would want his care to be individualized to reflect the unique God-made person he is.

Would you be surprised to learn that you likely know of and have seen Mr. W? At least on television, that is. The patient "Mr. W" I have described over the course of this chapter is none other than Karol Wojtyla, also known as St. John Paul II.

I believe his story is a strong witness to how every life, every soul, is so essentially important. Parkinson's disease was just part of his story; it never defined him. It was something that unfortunately could not be cured, but he did not let it stop him from living his life. Rather, he courageously displayed his progressive debility and frailty publicly, on an international stage, and continued to teach, love, and serve. Although he taught about suffering by his writing and speaking, some of his best teaching came by the way he lived. This man—truly brilliant and effervescent, even when wrought by the advanced stages of this illness—taught us by example how to suffer well. As then-Cardinal Joseph Ratzinger testified, John Paul II helps the Church understand that "even age has a message, and suffering a dignity and a salvific force."

Thank you and please pray for us, St. John Paul II!

Chapter 2

PALLIATIVE MEDICINE AND HOSPICE 101

In this chapter, we will review the medical subspecialty fields of palliative care and hospice. I will explain their similarities and also how they are inherently different. I will provide insight into their care philosophies, the scope of their practice, and the ways they can be beneficial. Throughout the chapter I will also be working to clarify several common misperceptions of palliative care and hospice. I will close by describing the special subset called perinatal palliative care and when it can be helpful.

MEET JOHN

John is a fifty-five-year-old gentleman who recently received a diagnosis of locally advanced pancreatic cancer. This is a very serious diagnosis. A small minority can be cured with aggressive treatment, but the majority will succumb to the disease. John and his wife of thirty years, Rose, are devastated by this news and want to take the most aggressive course of treatment to try to help John live as long as he can. They have four children who they shared are the "lights of our lives" and are expecting their first grandchild in six months. John's cancer doctor offers him chemotherapy and, if responsive, the possibility of surgery. The oncologist is honest about the challenges that John faces. John wants to fight.

WHAT IS PALLIATIVE CARE?

Reading the patient John's story, you may be thinking that it sounds like he is starting on a rough road. We want to work toward John's goals, and we want for him and his family to be well-supported and to be best prepared for whatever lies ahead. For anyone in a similar situation to John, I would want them to know about the field of palliative care, as it could well be of meaningful benefit to them.

Do not feel bad if you do not know what palliative care is—I definitely had not heard of the term growing up. When I learned what it was and began discerning that I would specialize in it, I realized I had to help others around me even pronounce it right! (It is pronounced "pal-lee-uh-tiv," in case you were wondering.) It comes from the root word *pallium*, meaning "to cloak." Not only that, there is a Catholic connection too. Who wears a pallium? The pope![1]

When you think about palliative care, think about "cloaking with support" someone who is going through a serious and difficult medical situation. The aim is to cloak them from all sides and to address all the aspects of their life that may be affected by the stress of the illness. The Center to Advance Palliative Medicine defines it as follows:

> Palliative care is specialized medical care for people living with a serious illness. This type of care is focused on providing relief from the symptoms and stress of the illness. The goal is to improve quality of life for both the patient and the family. Palliative care is provided by a specially-trained team of doctors, nurses and other specialists who work together with a patient's other doctors to provide an extra layer of support. Palliative care is based on the needs of the patient, not on the patient's prognosis. It is appropriate at any age and at any stage in a serious illness, and it can be provided along with curative treatment.[2]

To break this down a bit, palliative care—or the medical subspecialty of palliative medicine—is a specialty field like oncology or cardiology.

Physicians must obtain special yearlong fellowship training in addition to their general studies. This means that after choosing a field of medicine such as pediatrics, family practice, or internal medicine (adult care), they then choose to specialize in caring for patients with serious illness. During this year of additional studies, the physician learns special skills in symptom management, pain control, communication in challenging situations, and other issues related to the stresses associated with serious illness. The physician learns how to manage issues commonly associated with many different serious illnesses: dementia, heart failure, chronic obstructive pulmonary disease (COPD), cancer, kidney failure, liver failure, and more. The physician works to understand the stresses the patient is experiencing from the disease and from side effects of the treatment of the disease. These could range from physical symptoms to emotional stress to spiritual issues to financial and social distress.

Every doctor can help with communicating with patients and managing symptoms of their disease. These are considered "primary palliative care" skills. However, the more advanced training that a palliative medicine fellowship provides helps the physician go deeper and really hone "specialty palliative care" skills based on the best scientific evidence. For example, a primary care physician may be able to manage high blood pressure, but when heart stuff gets really complicated, the patient is referred to the heart specialist, a cardiologist. This is the same way it works with a palliative care specialist.

My palliative medicine fellowship truly provided a new perspective and philosophy switch from how I had previously approached caring for patients. Having previously trained in internal medicine, my goal was often to help cure or treat a problem to make it a nonissue for the patient. Now, as a palliative medicine physician, I was caring for patients with illnesses that medicine often could not cure or make better. I was also more focused on looking at patients through the lens of their emotional, psychosocial, and spiritual health, in addition to their physical issues. I realized that a key point was that although a patient's illness may not be curable, the focus is on helping them live as well as possible for as long as possible. It is important to find out who the patient is beyond their disease and who and what are most important to them. What are their values, preferences, and beliefs? And how do those beliefs get translated into their medical situation and decisions? The goal, I like to say, is to help promote and ensure "value-concordant" care.

As stress in serious illness can manifest in a variety of ways, what is neat about palliative care is that multiple disciplines often work together to give the patient and their family the best support. As a physician, I am often supported by palliative care nurses, social workers, and chaplains on my team. We all unite our strengths to help not only the patient but also all the people who love the patient. The patient's caregiver, family, friends, and greater community are all affected by this person's serious illness, and it is important to address their needs and concerns too.

Some Misconceptions

I have heard people say, when someone is getting palliative care, that it is a bad sign and that if they are "going palliative," the doctors have given up on them. This is incorrect. Adding palliative care to your medical team is supplying an additional layer of support to the team you already have. It is important to note that if you or your loved one gets a palliative care team, nothing—I repeat, *nothing*—is taken away from your other medical care. Palliative care only adds; it does not take anything away. You just get an added layer of support from a team of people whose aim is for you to live the best life you can despite this serious health issue. You will still have your other medical doctors to care for you, and you can continue with any and all current treatments you are receiving. If you have cancer and are receiving treatment with chemotherapy and radiation, that will continue. If you need medical care like hospitalization, blood transfusion, dialysis, surgery—all these things continue as before. It is erroneous to think that it is a bad sign (or sign of weakness) that you have palliative care. There should be no stigma associated with it. Is your health causing you or your family stress? Would you like the assistance of a team of people who are professionally trained to help manage that stress? If so, palliative care is for you!

Anytime that the additional support of a palliative care team could be helpful, I would encourage it. A landmark medical study that helped put palliative care on the map demonstrated that people are actually living longer when they have palliative care support than when they do not.[3] Having palliative care involved is just like having another type of specialty care medical doctor (such as your cancer specialist or kidney specialist) taking care of you. Their focus is not on a particular part of you, but instead they pay attention to how you are coping with your illness overall and offer ways that stress can be decreased. Your palliative care team should want to listen to you and understand who you are as a person and what you hold important. They are meant to be in your corner. If your goal is curing your illness and lengthening your life, that is their goal for you too. They may have honest conversations with you that discuss serious topics, but the aim of these is to ensure that you understand your medical situation and that they understand you.

Some people feel that anyone over a certain age should be receiving palliative care. This is also wrong thinking and makes me think of my dear great aunt, who is over one hundred years old. For someone of her advanced age, she is very healthy. Although she has developed some memory and functional losses from dementia, she does not have other medical diagnoses and does not take a lot of medications. She walks, visits with family, participates in social activities at her nursing home, and, most importantly, enjoys ice cream. She does not have a need for palliative care or hospice services. If she was sent to me as a patient consultation, I would even say she does not qualify for services. She does not have a serious illness, and old age does not qualify her. I would say, "Keep on eating ice cream!"

Someone's age does not denote whether they are appropriate for palliative care services. Someone's eligibility has much more to do with whether they have a serious illness and have associated stress, symptoms, and side effects. For my great aunt, if she has some significant health issue arise, she may well benefit from palliative care or hospice. It would be the same if she developed a kidney or heart problem and needed to see a specialist for those things. But in the meantime, with her stability, she is doing well and has no further need.

Benefits of Palliative Care

Palliative care can be helpful at any point in a serious illness: at the time of diagnosis, at a time when the disease progresses, at a time when there is a big decision to be made about care options, when the stresses of the illness seem to be a bit overwhelming, or just whenever the additional support could come in handy. For example, a patient with advanced multiple sclerosis was doing okay, but their spouse had a stroke and now cannot care for them in the same way—this would be a reasonable time for palliative care involvement. Or a patient's brain cancer was managed well with chemotherapy and the patient was in remission, but recent scans show the disease is back with a vengeance and causing debility. For some diseases (like particularly aggressive cancers) a referral to palliative care (to co-manage along with the other doctors) is recommended as standard practice of care. Palliative care has been proven to be of such meaningful benefit to these patients that it is considered a detriment when it is not part of their care.

Studies demonstrate that most people get palliative care services much later than they could, thereby not receiving the full benefit of the services. I think this has to do with the unfortunate stigma that continues to pervade popular understanding: that palliative care is for the end of life and therefore something to push off until absolutely necessary. Do not have fear! Palliative care is here for increased support and better management of the stresses caused by illness.

There are many ways that palliative care can help. What you may be able to expect from a consultation with a palliative care team may include medications to help with pain or other symptoms of the disease or side effects of treatment. The palliative care team could connect the patient and their family with community resources that could be helpful. Palliative care provides opportunities for clarification of the medical situation and care options, and it can solidify the patient's goals for their healthcare and life in the midst of this serious illness. Palliative care can help with things like advance directives and discussion about cardiac resuscitation ("do not resuscitate") options. The team can provide multidisciplinary support and has access to a chaplain who is trained to help with any spiritual stresses the patient may be experiencing. If there are any conflicts between the patient, their family, and their medical team, the palliative care team can also conduct meetings to help get everyone on the same page. The services can truly be helpful, and getting access to these sooner rather than later can often impart much more peace and assistance than anticipated.

Something many people are surprised to hear is that palliative care is not limited to any particular age: there is palliative care for children, adolescents, adults, and the elderly. There is even something called perinatal palliative care to help parents and families when they learn that their baby in utero has a serious or life-limiting diagnosis (see the next subsection of this chapter). Unfortunately, a reality of life is that serious illness can strike any person at any age and cause much havoc in their life and that of their family. It is particularly heartbreaking to see a child, adolescent, or young adult having to face a serious illness, and it is important to know that palliative care services are available for them too.

Pediatric palliative care is a growing field, and there are particular training programs for doctors to specialize in this. In my adult palliative care training fellowship, I spent a rotation at the local children's hospital, and it was a wonderful experience. Pediatric palliative care can be very helpful in places like the neonatal intensive care unit, helping support families of babies with rare and life-limiting genetic disorders, babies who had birth complications, or babies born premature. The team can help support children with cancers, neurological conditions, and developmental delays. They can help families of children who had been in serious accidents or had sustained trauma. In all these situations there are creative ways to provide developmentally and age-appropriate education and support for children and their siblings through the masterful work of Child Life Specialists. It is a great field to know about.

I like to say that in palliative care we "care for the patient and everyone who loves the patient." If someone you know with serious illness has young children or grandchildren in their life who may be struggling through this reality, encourage the patient to look into special resources for these important people. Whether through their medical team or palliative or hospice care, getting good, age-appropriate support can make a big difference, and it is important to inquire as to whether there are resources available (there likely are!).

Like other fields in healthcare, palliative care can be delivered in a variety of clinical settings. You can receive palliative care in the hospital setting, it can be embedded in specialty clinics (I have specifically seen this in heart failure, kidney failure, and cancer clinics), it can be independent in out-patient clinic settings, or it can be home-based, where a palliative team member comes to the patient's home.

WHAT IS PERINATAL PALLIATIVE CARE AND HOW DOES IT SUPPORT PATIENTS AND FAMILIES?

Did you know that palliative care services are even available for babies in utero? Well, palliative care is truly a "womb-to-tomb" kind of care! As much as we would not like to admit it, not every pregnancy goes smoothly, full of bliss and joy. Sadly, there are times when a couple may learn their baby has a life-limiting condition. With today's medical technology—ul-trasounds, genetic studies, and other testing—devastating conditions can be diagnosed much earlier. Although this news may lead some to terminate the pregnancy, for Catholics who acknowledge that life begins at concep-tion the field of perinatal palliative care can be a beautiful resource to sup-port with reverence the dignity of their baby's life.

The perinatal palliative care team works to support the family, coming up with the best birth plan to honor and aid them so they can love and pro-mote the dignity of their baby in the best way possible. A perinatal pallia-tive care team will work to aid the baby's parents and other family members to best prepare for cherishing the baby for as long as God naturally wills them to live. Prior to birth, the team can meet to create a birth plan that may focus on comfort and calm (instead of frenetic beeping machines that cannot fix or cure) and incorporate things like the Sacrament of Baptism from a priest, time for family members to be present, music, and lega-cy-building and memory-making activities such as taking handprints and footprints. Perinatal palliative care can help make the life of the newborn, as limited as it may be, rich, meaningful, and special. They work to provide opportunities for parents to be parents and siblings to be siblings, and as sad as the situation is, this experience can be very healing and beautiful and provide much aid in the grieving process.

In my experience, the family's obstetrical doctors will be able to connect the family with perinatal palliative support and will know when it would be beneficial. If something happens unexpectedly with a preterm labor or birth, the neonatal intensive care team can also connect family with palliative services.

WHAT IS HOSPICE CARE?

It is important to realize that palliative care and hospice are not synonymous terms. Often the terms are used interchangeably, and that is incorrect. Actually, one of the takeaways I hope you glean from reading this book is that palliative care and hospice each have a unique purpose and place in healthcare. The way you should think about it is that hospice is a *type* of palliative care; hospice falls under the bigger umbrella of palliative care (and definitely not all palliative care is hospice).

To explain further the difference between palliative care and hospice, let us return to John—the patient we were introduced to at the beginning of the chapter who is dealing with a new diagnosis of locally advanced pancreatic cancer—using this graphic to assist us.

SUPPORT IN ADVANCED ILLNESS: PALLIATIVE CARE AND HOSPICE

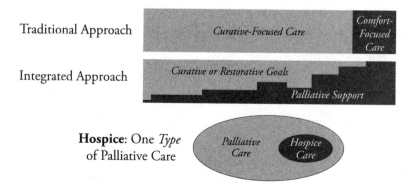

Traditional Approach — Curative-Focused Care — Comfort-Focused Care

Integrated Approach — Curative or Restorative Goals — Palliative Support

Hospice: One *Type* of Palliative Care — Palliative Care — Hospice Care

John is starting his cancer journey with a plan for aggressive care and a desire for life-prolonging treatments. Let's place him on the top bar in this graphic, the "traditional approach" to care. He begins his treatments, the curative-focused care part of the graph. At some point along the way, John's cancer grows, despite the treatment. He gets switched to another kind of chemotherapy. He develops some related pain and nausea. He keeps pushing ahead. Despite everything, John gets very ill and cannot tolerate the treatment well. He is hospitalized and is quite debilitated. His cancer doctor visits him and says, "John, there is nothing more we can do." The cancer has progressed and there is no effective treatment to combat it. It is time to focus on John's comfort, as his death is likely near.

Reading John's situation may come across as a bit jarring. It is meant to. If his health was compared to driving a car, it may seem like having the foot on the gas, even "flooring it," all along the curative-focused care area of the top bar on the graph. And then, all of a sudden, the foot is slammed on the brake. The car comes to a complete stop. There is a sense of bewilderment; there can also be a sense of abandonment, of having expectations not met, and of much grief as the switch is made to the comfort-focused care part of the graph.

Alternatively, let's say that right from the beginning, after John has received his diagnosis, he is introduced to palliative care. This correlates with the second bar, the "integrated approach" to care. John is referred to meet with the palliative team (the palliative support part of the bar graph). His goal is the same: to aggressively pursue disease-directed treatments to fight his cancer. Initially he may not need the palliative care team much (and the palliative support area of the graph is comparatively small). John is focused on the chemotherapy. Yet, at some point along the way, John, like many patients, may begin to experience some physical symptoms related to his cancer, like abdominal pain or nausea. He may worry about how to talk about his diagnosis with his kids. He may not be sleeping as well and be struggling with some worries about the future. These are all ways the palliative care team can help John.

As time goes on, John works with both his cancer team and his palliative team. Scans show that his cancer is growing despite the treatments. He switches to try a new type of chemotherapy. He gets weaker. He is admitted to the hospital. The palliative care team continues to support him, and he visits with them regularly and finds their assistance meaningful and beneficial to his care (the palliative support area grows some on the graph). His first grandchild is born, and he enjoys holding the baby. Another of his goals has been to walk his daughter down the aisle at her wedding, and he does this. A month later scans again show the cancer is not responding as hoped to the treatment. After more conversations with his cancer doctor and the palliative care team, John decides that rather than continuing the battle to fight his cancer, which is a fight he knows he will ultimately not win, it would be better to pivot. Now the best fight is the battle for good days and being home with his family. He does not want to spend more time at the hospital, away from them. John is a fighter and he keeps fighting for this. He wants medications to keep his symptoms managed and to live the best life he can for as long as he can, realizing that at some point he will die of the cancer.

It is at this time that palliative care transitions to hospice care. Earlier in the process, hospice would not have been appropriate. But at this point, hospice is the subtype of palliative care that is most consistent with his goals and would most benefit him. With good and honest communication all along the way, this transition from palliative care to hospice should be seamless and peaceful for John and his family.

When It Is Time for Hospice

Hospice at its most basic is a Medicare benefit that covers medical care for patients who have been deemed by two physicians to have an estimation of six months or less to live due to a terminal diagnosis. But let us unpack this a bit further.

For hospice to make sense, a patient must have two things. One, they must have a diagnosis that qualifies them for hospice services (there are Medicare guidelines that a patient must meet—essentially that they have a serious, life-limiting diagnosis). Two, they must decide to no longer pursue disease-directed care and desire more of a comfort, symptoms-focused approach to their medical care. So a patient must have a diagnosis and also agree with the hospice philosophy. Without both, hospice does not make sense and is not the right choice for a patient.

If a patient and their family feels their goals of care are consistent with the hospice care philosophy (ready to transition to a comfort-based rather than disease-directed care, preferring to spend time at home rather than at the hospital), after speaking with the patient's physicians, it can be appropriate to have a hospice evaluation, where the hospice team will assess whether a patient qualifies for services. Most often, if a patient is in this kind of situation, they clearly do. A scenario where I have seen a patient not be eligible for hospice is someone with dementia who has some cognitive limitations and behavioral problems but is still otherwise healthy and able to do some things for themselves. This situation is often very stressful for caregivers, but the patient may not yet be in the advanced stages of illness or close to the end of life and therefore not meet Medicare guidelines.

The hospice Medicare benefit includes medical care given by the hospice team, medications (often delivered to where the patient is—not needing to be picked up at a pharmacy by the patient's family), and any medical equipment that may be helpful (such as a hospital bed, bedside toilet, or portable oxygen). These things are free to the patient, which is often a big relief to them and their family. The hospice benefit does not cover room and board for where a patient lives (like nursing home costs). The hospice team will work with the patient and family to creatively figure out a safe and feasible living situation, a conversation often assisted by the social worker. The majority of patients on hospice live in their own home or the home of a family member or friend, cared for by loved ones.

I have encountered some patients who believe that a person is only eligible for six months of hospice care and so they must wait to use this aid until they really need it. This is not true. If you are eligible for hospice services, you can be enrolled. Every few months you will be re-evaluated to ensure you still qualify for services, but if you do, the care will continue. I have taken care of patients who have been on hospice care services for years!

In rare instances, a patient may be found to no longer be eligible for hospice services because their health has stabilized or improved. This can happen with the attentive care a hospice team provides! In these situations, a patient can "graduate" from hospice services and would likely benefit from continued palliative care support. The patient can be re-evaluated again in the future, should their health situation change. I most commonly see this situation arise in patients who have chronic frailty, with or without chronic medical conditions.

Studies show that most people get on hospice very close to the end of life, and this means that they may not get to take advantage of the many benefits the service offers. If you or your loved one is eligible for hospice and the care seems to be the right thing in your health situation, I recommend trying it—do not worry about saving up your "eligible days" until later. Hospice is not meant to be only for the very end of life. I regularly tell patients: Hospice is not here to help you die. Hospice is here to help you live until you naturally die. Hospice walks alongside you and supports your goals, trying to help you make each day the most comfortable and pleasant it can be, for as long as possible. Hospice is not something to wait for until you or a loved one is already near the time of death. If you take this approach, you and your family might miss out on so many of the helpful and meaningful resources that hospice has to offer (included for free with enrollment). In addition to physicians and nurses, hospice has chaplaincy, social work, volunteers, caregiver support, and respite care (where hospice actually will cover a number of days of free room and board every so often to allow the patient's caregiver an often much-needed break) that are all available but often underutilized. Enrolling in hospice "early enough" will allow a patient to benefit from the services while living their life with their goals in mind, often relieving many areas of previously high stress.

Specific Hospice Services

Hospice, as an extension of and similar to palliative care, provides a multi-disciplinary team approach focused on management of suffering and holistic, patient-focused care. Hospice is not a specific place where a patient must go, but is a philosophy of care that comes wherever the patient lives and where they want to be. It can occur in a variety of settings: a private home, an apartment, an assisted living facility, or a nursing home. Hospice can take place in a hospital if a patient is too sick or unstable to be transported elsewhere. I have even heard of hospice taking place in a homeless shelter when a patient does not have a stable place to live. It is important that patients get meaningful care where they are safe and, hopefully, where they want to be.

In some cases, a patient's symptoms or medical situation may require more around-the-clock supervision and care. In situations like this, having a patient actually go to an inpatient hospice center to receive care is meaningfully beneficial. Staffed by hospice nurses 24/7 and with daily visits from a hospice physician, an inpatient unit is a place where patients can get a higher-intensity level of care if needed. After a couple days of attentive medication management and frequent dose adjustments, patients can often return home with symptoms improved. Other times, a patient may remain at the hospice center through the end of life, but this is typically because death is imminent.

In my experience, inpatient hospice centers are peace-filled and very family-friendly. Patient rooms resemble a hotel more than a hospital, and there is usually a chapel and even a kitchen and living areas for family members. Often, patients even have private areas outside, like spacious patios. It can be a beautiful alternative to the home setting when the patient's symptoms and situation necessitate it.

Some people have a mindset that hospice is only for very elderly patients or those who have cancer. Although hospice is well-equipped to take care of these patient populations, it is important to know that their services extend well beyond them. Like general palliative care, hospice is available for people of any age. In some cities, there are special inpatient hospice units for pediatric or adolescent populations. Hospice teams are experts at managing the symptoms of the dying process of any diagnosis; they are definitely not limited to cancer alone.

Life with Hospice

Hospice team members make regular visits to the patient, so as to be attentive to their comfort and any concerning signs or symptoms of distress they may be experiencing. The team member who most frequently visits is the hospice nurse, who is in communication with the hospice physician overseeing the care. Hospice workers are not in the patient's home 24/7, but they are always available by phone. On hospice, patients hopefully are able to stay in their home, and if a health crisis occurs, hospice is called rather than 911.

With hospice, patients are encouraged to live as normal a life as they can, eating and doing what they want. Although the patient may now be forgoing medical treatments that they no longer feel are beneficial, they are continued on medications that help them feel better. The hospice team's aim, like palliative care's, is to live the best life possible for as long as possible. Although the hospice team will care for a patient through the end of their earthly life, the dying itself is only a small part of what the service encompasses. Hospice's job is to walk with seriously ill patients and support them and their families all along their illness until the time of their natural death. Hospice is about helping families treasure this time and making it as smooth and full of meaning as possible. It is not at all about hastening a patient's dying process.

I must sadly admit that I have heard many stories of families feeling that their loved one's death was actively hastened by hospice. Given my experience, I acknowledge this could be possible, but I imagine most cases are due to suboptimal communication between the hospice team and family. If the reasons behind providing or discontinuing care and medications were well explained along the way by the hospice team, and if the family honestly shared their questions and any concerns, I feel the situations would have been greatly improved. This being said, if you ever have concerns about anything the hospice team is doing or not doing, do not hesitate to bring it up to your hospice team. You deserve good explanations. If you are ever not reassured or cannot get your concerns addressed, consider seeking a different hospice agency that will communicate better. This is already a stressful time; you need to feel peaceful about the care of your hospice team. I also encourage you to be very open about the patient's values and preferences. For example, for Catholics, telling the hospice team about the value one places on their faith, respect for the dignity of life, and so forth (the principles we discuss in this book!) would always be worthwhile.

It is also important to note that consenting to hospice services does not mean you are "locked in"; hospice is not a dead-end road. If you or your loved one enrolls in hospice, at any point you can discontinue it and transition back to your previous care (which would mean going to the hospital, getting aggressive medical treatments, etc.). Hospice is meant to be helpful and align with what you want for your life. If it does not, then hospice is not meant for you.

A scenario I commonly come across is that a patient on hospice will experience something like a fall that breaks their hip. Fixing the hip with orthopedic surgery would be greatly helpful, not to mention that it would likely improve their discomfort quite a bit! What is often the best plan is to discontinue hospice services, get admitted to the hospital for hip surgery, and then postoperatively decide whether to go back on hospice. Often, it makes sense to resume services, but in some cases it does not. Just remember, hospice is a free choice that is meant to be helpful. It is never something you are locked into.

DO PALLIATIVE CARE AND HOSPICE MEAN GIVING UP ON LIFE?

No, definitely not. Again, palliative care is an *extra layer* of support when you are going through a serious illness. In my mind, you are even more intensely digging into life, to living the best life you can despite your illness. This view is supported by the previously mentioned article (by Jennifer Temel and others) that pointed to the benefits of palliative care.[4] In the study, researchers looked at patients with advanced lung cancer. The patients were split into two groups. In group one, the patients received what they called "standard" oncologic (cancer) care, following their oncologist and receiving available treatments. In group two, the patients received standard oncologic care and also palliative care. Guess what the results were. The patients in group two who had palliative care lived significantly longer! They also spent less time in the hospital, which generally is not where a patient wants to be. This article also demonstrated that getting palliative care involved early in the disease journey can provide more meaningful benefits than waiting until much later.

And when a patient and their family decide that it is time to transition to hospice care, that is not giving up either. As mentioned before, it is just reframing the situation from fighting *against the disease* to fighting *for good days* with comfort, most often surrounded by loved ones.

If we think back to John, the patient with pancreatic cancer, his primary goal with his cancer treatment was to help him live longer so as to be around for his family. And that was the palliative care team's goal for him too. When his cancer progressed despite trying different kinds of treatment and his disease symptoms and treatment side effects were causing him to be hospitalized, forcing him to spend more time away from the people he loved, he discerned how he might need to pivot his fight and best meet his goals another way. By having hospice care come to his house and focus on his physical comfort and mental clarity (and emotional and spiritual support as well!), he would get more time with family and feel better while he was with them. He was still fighting for this precious time with loved ones, and hospice was helping to support this.

HOW DO PALLIATIVE CARE AND HOSPICE HELP RELIEVE STRESS IN SERIOUS ILLNESS?

As anyone can attest, it is no fun getting sick. Add to that an illness that is quite debilitating, possibly incurable, and significantly affects one's functioning in daily life. Stress presents in so many forms in a serious illness and is very specific to each individual patient. Dame Cicely Saunders, MD, a founder of hospice and palliative care, used the term "total pain" to describe all the encompassing physical, emotional, spiritual, and social stress that is experienced by patients going through a serious illness. One aspect of a patient's pain cannot be adequately addressed when others are ignored. It is only through looking at all the symptoms and stresses in total that progress toward comfort and healing can be achieved. We will now briefly touch on several domains of stress and suffering that palliative care and hospice work to improve.

Often stress in serious illness comes in the form of physical pain, distressing symptoms, or bothersome side effects of treatment. As a palliative care physician, I work to address pain management needs and received special training on how to do this safely and effectively. Other common physical issues in serious illness that I work to address include shortness of breath, nausea, constipation, diarrhea, poor appetite, fatigue, and insomnia. I consider lifestyle modifications or other medications that may help. Often, I use medications for their side effects: for a cancer patient who is feeling depressed, for example, I may consider a medication that not only can help improve the patient's mood but can also improve appetite and sleep. Although weight gain and feeling sleepier are normally unattractive side effects of a medication for healthy people, for cancer patients who are losing weight unintentionally and struggling with getting restorative sleep these side effects are often welcome and helpful.

While physical stresses of illness may appear the most straightforward, stress most certainly does not end there. Serious illness can cause immense emotional impact. A patient may not be as functional as they previously were. Their body does not work the same—perhaps they have lost the ability to control their bowels or bladder. They are often not as mobile as they used to be and may feel less useful to others. They may even feel they are a "burden" to their family or caregiver. This can evolve into significant anger or resentment. There can be a sense that they are letting others down. Issues like depression and anxiety are very common. Serious illness can also bring about more interpersonal conflicts as unresolved issues from the past, or other difficult conflicts, can rise to the surface. Sometimes a disease brings out the best in a patient's loved ones, but sometimes it can bring to light the worst.

A serious illness can also include much social suffering. For, as it brings forth much potential change in a patient's life, it can often cause change in that patient's roles in their family, community, and workplace. For many patients with a serious illness, they are no longer able to work, or must significantly scale back. This may cause them much disappointment, as they previously defined themselves by this work and their associated achievements. There can also be much isolation related to a serious illness. Sometimes patients feel quite embarrassed when the disease or treatment changes their physical appearance. They may lose their hair or gain or lose a lot of weight. They may just feel they look "sick." This can impact their willingness to participate in social events, even if they feel up to it physically. There is much loss patients can experience with this, not to mention the challenge of being unable to fulfill commitments they previously held as important. They can feel quite isolated from their family, friends, and community and that they can no longer relate to others. It is exhausting to share about one's illness over and over again, and even if others can understand or relate in some way and honestly want to meaningfully help, they may not quite know how.

A serious illness can also significantly impact patients financially. I will admit that this is an area I received little training in. However, it is so important that I acknowledge patients' financial concerns if I am to help them holistically. Often, this concern can be expressed by merely raising the issue with a comment such as the following: "For many people in situations similar to yours, they feel stressed around financial concerns and unknowns. I am curious if these issues are affecting you at all." Most often, patients heave a big sigh of relief and emphatically say, "Yes!" Navigating the healthcare system can be so overwhelming, even more so during a serious illness. Most people have never planned for something like this. Their plans for their life were so different. It is not uncommon for people to use their savings for healthcare costs, to face the loss of home or property, to face the prospect of leaving significant debt behind to others, to face losing their independence and needing a higher level of care in a facility, and to face many insurance complexities. The palliative care team social worker can be of particular help to patients and families with these concerns and can help direct them to other community resources and programs.

Spiritual and existential distress can also be a huge (and too often unspoken) area of significant pain and suffering for patients. These are not necessarily specifically religious issues. Of course, religious issues can arise and are important to address, but what I am more speaking about here are issues related to meaning, identity, and personal value, which for the patient have been affected by the disease. Sometimes a disease causes a patient to feel that their integrity as a person has been compromised. It is a very deep suffering that can impact their ability to believe and trust others or to connect with their loved ones or the healthcare team. It can cause a lack of peace and bring up other unresolved issues in their life. It can ultimately lead them to request hastening the end of their life and to consider things like physician-assisted suicide or euthanasia.

As a palliative care physician, seeing a patient in any kind of distress can be heart-wrenching, but seeing someone suffer from spiritual and existential distress is in my opinion the hardest. It at times feels so intimidating to work to address this, and I feel my training in this area has been inadequate. Despite this, I believe that it is even more imperative that I do not shy away from addressing this distress when I see it. By imploring the Holy Spirit's assistance, I must patiently and lovingly accompany patients through this and work in any way I can to restore their integrity and help them see their dignity and worth. I also greatly appreciate the expertise of chaplains who can provide much meaningful support to a patient and family experiencing spiritual or existential distress, as well as to the palliative care team. By addressing a patient's "total pain," the palliative care or hospice team can take an effective and individualized approach to meaningfully decrease a patient's suffering.

I would be remiss if I did not note that the stress of a serious illness does not affect only the patients themselves. It extends to all the people who love them, particularly their caregivers. Evidence shows that the health of a patient's caregiver decreases when they are busy caring for their loved one. They just do not have time to go to the dentist or eye doctor and get those yearly checkups like they should! Particularly in caregivers of dementia patients, the care can take quite an emotional, physical, and spiritual toll.[5] As I mentioned earlier, in palliative care we say, "We take care of the patient and everyone who loves the patient." Team members take particular notice to support the caregiver and to provide them the personal care and attention they need.

It is important to know that this care does not end with the patient's death. The patient's loved ones are eligible for free grief counseling and bereavement services, usually through the first anniversary of the patient's death. Particularly when a death may be very sudden, unexpected, traumatic, or involving the loss of a young adult or child, I strongly recommend that families at least be made aware of these resources. Palliative care teams can also help patients and families work through anticipatory grief, grieving the loss before it even occurs.

This chapter covered many aspects of the fields of palliative medicine and hospice care. My aim was to help explain the scope of the field and provide answers to many common questions and address common misunderstandings I see. With this framework, we will proceed to more specific issues in the remainder of this book.

Chapter 3

COMMUNICATION AROUND SERIOUS ILLNESS

This chapter's aim is to help increase your confidence around honestly sharing any concerns you may have with your doctors and medical team. It is important to ask your questions, and I will provide information and encouragement about ways to successfully advocate for yourself and your loved ones. We will also review how Catholic ethical teaching is applied and helps guide making healthcare decisions. In addition, I will share practical guidance on how to discuss your medical situation and your preferences regarding your care with your loved ones. Although this can all sound quite daunting, we will work to approach it with less stress and more peace. Let us start by learning about two patients who are quite different, but have a similar serious medical issue.

MEET ELIZABETH AND JOSEPH

Elizabeth is a forty-year-old woman, otherwise healthy, who has a genetic kidney condition (polycystic kidney disease). She is married, is a mother of two young children, and works part-time at a local hair salon. She has been followed by a nephrologist (kidney specialist) for years and, despite their best efforts, her kidney failure has progressed to the point of needing dialysis.

Joseph is an eighty-year-old gentleman with advanced dementia and hearing and vision loss, who lives at a nursing facility and has advanced heart disease that is affecting his kidneys.

He has a hard time recognizing his family these days but enjoys being around people. His doctor recently shared with his family that his kidney failure has progressed to the point of needing dialysis.

IF I AM DIAGNOSED WITH A SERIOUS ILLNESS, WHAT KINDS OF QUESTIONS SHOULD I BE ASKING MY DOCTOR?

The patients Elizabeth and Joseph each have a big medical decision to make. They have kidney failure and are now being confronted with whether or not to pursue dialysis. For anyone with a serious illness, it can feel simply overwhelming thinking about all the unknowns. Your mind may be buzzing around, and it may be challenging to focus. There are so many stresses and so many questions. It seems as if after the doctor said the word "cancer" or "heart failure" or "dementia," you lost track of everything else he was saying. Your thoughts go to someone you know with a similar diagnosis, or you start thinking about all the affairs you now urgently feel the need to get in order. How are you going to tell your kids? How will you financially afford the needed healthcare? Before you know it, the doctor is leaving the room and you do not feel like you understand anything!

With the myriad of thoughts and stresses like those detailed above, it is not uncommon that what a patient understands is different from what the doctor believes they comprehend. I cannot tell you the number of times I have read in a patient's chart that their cancer is incurable and that this has been explained to them. The treatments being offered are not meant to cure but are aiming at keeping the cancer from growing as fast or spreading to other places in the body. However, when I ask the patient to tell me what they understand about their medical situation, they tell me their doctor is working to help cure them and they are expecting the cancer to all go away. It is clear that the patient and the doctor are not on the same page. This is no one's fault, but it is a major source of miscommunication.

It is unfortunate when I learn of this discrepancy in understanding, and I feel sad for the patient. I do not want to take away their hope by clarifying the reality of the situation for them, but it is also important that they know the truth. If I gently and kindly rectify any points of misunderstanding, this knowledge can empower a patient. Many times, a person may choose to live their life a bit differently based on their prognosis. For, if you knew you had a limited life expectancy of months to years, would you take a different approach to your life? I imagine I would.

Oftentimes, it is on a follow-up medical visit that you will have had more time to process what was previously told to you, gather your thoughts, formulate your questions (I recommend writing them down), and may even bring a friend or family member with you as a "second set of ears" to listen and help advocate for you. Sometimes it is not even your primary doctor, but another doctor—perhaps on the palliative care team—who can take the time to sit with you and sort out your questions and concerns. It is essential that your questions are answered so that you can feel peaceful about the plan ahead. I have included a list of common good questions to ask, which will help empower you to obtain the information you need to make the best medical decisions. As difficult as asking some of these questions may be, I believe knowledge is power, and you need to know and understand what the doctors know and understand about your diagnosis, prognosis, and treatment options.

- Can you further explain the type of disease I have, and what is the current stage and grade? What do these terms mean?
- What is the expected course of my disease? What can you tell me about my prognosis?
- Is it reversible? Is it curable?
- If not, can my life be extended? By what means, and how successful is that for people in my condition?
- How long can I expect that extension to continue?
- What treatment options are available? Are there significant side effects?
- Does this treatment cure me, change the course of the disease, or slow it down?

- What is the meaningful benefit of these treatments in my case—what would you most recommend?
- What would success look like?
- What percentage of patients like me get better from this treatment, and for how long?
- Will this treatment help me be more active in the future?
- Will it make me more comfortable in the future?
- When can I expect to feel some results?
- What is the best way to communicate with my medical team if I have issues with the treatment or other problems?
- What lifestyle changes should I consider?
- Is this condition genetic? Should I have other members of my family go through any testing or screening for this?
- Can you recommend some other reliable resources (printed or on-line) for learning more about my diagnosis?
- Are there any clinical trials for my condition? If so, do you have access to these trials?
- Would a palliative care consultation, to work with you on managing my symptoms, be helpful? Is there a palliative care physician you've worked with? (For information about palliative care, go to: http://www.getpalliativecare.org/download/GetPCHandout.pdf)
- When will I have results, and will you call me?[1]

HOW DO I APPROACH WEIGHING WHICH HEALTHCARE OPTIONS ARE BEST FOR ME?

At some point in your healthcare journey, you or your loved one may be offered a treatment that is in the category of what I will call "advanced medical technology." At its most basic level, these kinds of treatments come up in serious illness and often help prolong life through "artificial" means. They help your body function more normally. They are, in a sense, "life support." None of these medical interventions can provide a cure to the underlying problem. They help provide immediate stabilization and regulation. They are life-sustaining treatments (as your body may cease to function without them). Sometimes the technology can be helpful temporarily, to help one get over the hump of an exacerbation of illness and get back to a previous state of health. Other times, the technology may be meant for longer-term use, or even considered for use for the rest of someone's life.

I am referring to technology like dialysis machines, which our two patients we met at the beginning of the chapter, Elizabeth and Joseph, were thinking about starting. But this is not just limited to dialysis—things like ventilator machine support, an organ transplant, a surgery, chemotherapy, and serial blood transfusions could also be challenging options to contemplate. Considering any one of these technologies can feel difficult or even overwhelming. It is important for us to realize that, as Catholics, the decision of whether or not to pursue an advanced medical technology is rarely black or white. But we do have meaningful guidance from the Church that is quite helpful in weighing our options in order to make decisions that align with our Catholic values and beliefs.

And these decisions can be complicated to process! We have a desire to live as well as we can. Yet, while we are seeking this best life, at the same time we cannot cling to life unrealistically. For we are not meant to be "vitalists," required to utilize every available means to preserve life simply because it is possible or offered. As Catholics, we have a moral obligation to protect life, but not one to excessively prolong it.

At the same time, there exists the desire to die well, to die at the end of a life well-lived, to die a natural death. We are not meant to ignore the dignity of life, particularly when we cannot cure what afflicts us. How do we balance all of this?

You may have heard of the terms "ordinary" and "extraordinary" care. Ordinary care means that something is basic or necessary. As Catholics, we are obligated to pursue ordinary care. Extraordinary care is considered more exceptional, or optional, and not necessarily a treatment you need to choose. However, the Church has actually provided other terms that can be even more helpful in discernment. These are "proportionate" and "disproportionate." Think again of a balancing scale here, where on one side you have all the benefits of a treatment and, on the other, the burdens. A key important point here is that we look at everything through the perspective of the patient, which is the determinant of what is burdensome or beneficial. Proportionate care, in the eyes of the patient, offers reasonable hope of benefit without imposing disproportionate burdens. Benefit in this case outweighs burden. Disproportionate care tips the scale the other way for the patient. If something is disproportionate, the care does *not* offer reasonable hope of benefit and *does* impose disproportionate burdens. Burden in this case outweighs benefit.

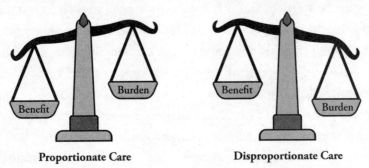

Proportionate Care   **Disproportionate Care**

When determining whether a treatment option is proportionate or disproportionate, it is important to think about questions such as "What good can this treatment do *for* this person I love?" and "What harm can it do *to* him or her?" The same treatment option may be proportionate for one person and disproportionate to the next. Even for the same person, a treatment option may at some point in time be proportionate and then at a later time be disproportionate.

In general, if a treatment is clearly proportionate, it should be pursued. If a treatment is seeming more disproportionate, it can be declined. Declining something that is disproportionate is not immoral and is not the equivalent of giving up or committing suicide.

It is essential to have clear communication with your healthcare team about the risks, benefits, alternative options, and potential consequences of proceeding with or abstaining from a treatment. It is important that the option in question is fully understood. You need to ensure you have all the information necessary to make the most informed and best decision. Just because something *can* be offered does not mean it necessarily *should*. Put the option on the scale, and see how it balances out.

The decision-making involved here, as you may imagine, depends on the context for each patient and is individualized, as each person's situation is different. Take the two patients Elizabeth and Joseph introduced at the beginning of the chapter who are both dealing with kidney failure and considering dialysis.

Although Elizabeth and Joseph each has the same decision before them, it is clear that the contexts of their individual situations are quite different. Elizabeth is forty years old, is a caregiver to two children, and has no other medical problems, while Joseph is eighty years old, is dependent upon care from others, and has many health limitations from his advanced dementia and heart disease.

Starting dialysis treatment would likely mean going to a dialysis center for four hours at a time, three times a week. It would also mean getting a special IV line to get the treatment, unless the patient has prepared their blood vessels by a special surgery to create something called a fistula in their arm.

Let us apply the concepts I explained earlier. Does dialysis for one of these patients seem more proportionate than it does for the other? It would be important to know, particularly for Joseph, if there were any current or previously expressed wishes or desires regarding dialysis. It is important also to consider what good or harm dialysis could do for each patient. You can see how this process of discernment is quite individualized and how dialysis would look different for each person. If one of the patients deems dialysis proportionate and starts the treatment, the scale balancing benefit and burden should continue to be considered as they proceed with dialysis. For at some time in the future, if the scale begins to tip and the treatment brings what is considered more burden than benefit (for example, the patient continues to experience complications from dialysis like infections or blood pressure problems, or other organ systems start to fail), the treatment should again be evaluated. If the dialysis truly becomes disproportionate at some point in time, in that situation it can be appropriate to consider discontinuation.

HOW DO I HAVE CONVERSATIONS WITH MY FAMILY ABOUT MY HEALTHCARE PREFERENCES?

Reading this book and thinking through these topics is difficult enough. It is a whole other level to discuss these issues with loved ones. The truth is, everyone comes to conversations like this from a different perspective and framework. It is often uncomfortable to speak about healthcare preferences with our loved ones because, well, we love them! We do not want to consider that they may become sick one day (or learn they already are dealing with something). We may feel that having these conversations may burden our loved ones in some way. Yet, I can confidently say from my medical and personal experience that these conversations are so important. For your loved ones to learn what you honestly feel about your preferences is truly a gift to them.

As far as practical tips to have a successful conversation, I would definitely provide a "warning shot"—it is most certainly preferable to prepare others that you want to talk about your health or potential issues down the road rather than springing the conversation on them unexpectedly. I would recommend finding a time where everyone can be calm, rested, and fully present. Do not try to tack this conversation on to a busy family dinner or holiday gathering where there are sure to be distractions. Be ready for questions and be patient with your loved ones, as you will likely have thought about this more and have more comfort discussing it than they have. I also would recommend saying a little silent prayer before starting, something like "Come, Holy Spirit," to help calm you and provide you wisdom and guidance on what and how you communicate.

There are some great tools out there to guide you in your discussion. "The Conversation Project" (https://theconversationproject.org) is one I encourage because it has helpful, practical, and free resources. It also has additional guides you can complete to help you best identify your values and what underpins your healthcare choices, which can be great preparation for these conversations. You can also, of course, decide to fill these out with your family present.

Another great resource is "Five Wishes" (https://www.fivewishes.org/for-myself/), which is a value-based guide to identifying your preferences. It includes some topics usually encompassed by advance directive documents. If you complete this, it can be very helpful to also share it with your medical team.

Sometimes a less daunting approach is to tell one trusted friend or family member about your health situation and invite them to join you for a doctor's appointment. Here, your physician can help explain things to them, and the situation will not just be in your own words. This person, now understanding things on the same page as you, can then be with you and help provide support as you share with others. Or, if you have a palliative care team, ask a member of their team to be with you as you share with your family. Do what you need to feel supported!

It may at times feel like the best thing to do with your medical situation is to keep everything to yourself. But in general, this is not something I recommend. Not only can this be a stressful and lonely path to tread, it does not offer your loved ones the opportunity to love and support you in a special way.

It takes courage and strength to have these important conversations, but I really recommend doing so. Your family may not realize it now, but I assure you, it is a true gift to know your preferences. Knowing how you feel about different healthcare choices will most certainly impart peace in the future around respecting your wishes. In the next couple of chapters, we will look at specific things you may choose to discuss and how you can best document your preferences in writing.

I believe you can do it. Be assured you are in my prayers.

Chapter 4

NAVIGATING TREATMENT OPTIONS

In this chapter, we will continue to explore Catholic ethical teaching and apply it to common and often difficult healthcare decisions. I will particularly highlight the issues around pain medication like opioids, artificial nutrition and hydration, mechanical ventilation, and dialysis.

MEET PHILIP

Philip is a seventy-two-year-old gentleman with colon cancer that has also spread to his liver and lungs. He is currently undergoing treatment for his cancer, which seems to be generally keeping the cancer at bay, and recent scans show it has not spread anywhere else. He lives with his wife, Anne, and they enjoy babysitting their grandchildren. Philip is also known for his meticulously kept lawn and his flower garden. Because of his cancer, he has developed significant pain in his abdomen that impairs his ability to sleep through the night and rest during the day. The pain is making it harder to help Anne babysit, and he recently had to get a lawn care service, for the first time in his life. He has tried over-the-counter pain relievers with no success and is worried about taking anything stronger as he wants to be as alert and active as possible and does not want to become addicted to anything.

ARE PAIN MEDICATIONS SAFE TO TAKE? DO THEY CAUSE BAD SIDE EFFECTS?

Philip has been diagnosed with a serious illness, colon cancer, and unfortunately has started having associated abdominal pain that is quite debilitating and affecting his everyday life. Like many people, he highly values being active and spending quality time with loved ones. And, of course, he values having mental clarity.

It is clear that Philip's pain symptoms need to be taken seriously and that at this point he warrants a stronger medication than can be obtained over the counter. Medically, it is reasonable to consider initiation of an opioid like morphine or oxycodone. This word may send up alarm signals—*an opioid?* Is Philip really that sick? Don't only dying patients get put on morphine? And then, are we not concerned that he will get addicted?

These are common questions and natural concerns about strong pain medications, and I shared these concerns when I started training. I, like many people, had a real case of "opiophobia" (the fear of opioids). I did not feel comfortable prescribing them, I felt anxious when I had patients who were on them, and I worried that when I prescribed them, patients would manipulate me and go try to sell them on the streets. In the course of my palliative medicine fellowship training, I received a lot of education about the correct and safe usages of opioids, particularly in the seriously ill. I learned that pain in the setting of serious illness is approached differently than acute pain after a surgery or chronic musculoskeletal pain from a remote injury. The standard of care for managing pain from cancer and other advanced illnesses is, in fact, opioids. It is like using insulin to treat someone with diabetes. If someone has cancer pain, you often manage it with opioids. In my work in palliative care, opioids are so frequently used because research has shown them to be effective for other, often debilitating symptoms common in serious illness. For example, opioids are the first-line recommended treatment for shortness of breath in advanced lung and heart disease (it is amazing the relief they provide!). They have also been found to be helpful with cough issues and anxiety related to other symptoms.

Starting an opioid on someone like Philip is, of course, not without its risks. Opioids are controlled substances that do have addictive potential, and it is important to manage them with safety protocols in place. Misuse or overdosing of opioids can lead to serious things like decreasing the drive to breathe (respiratory depression), which can have lethal consequences. There are many tools available to help physicians safely prescribe opioids. One is performing an opioid risk assessment. By assessing things such as the patient's family or personal history of substance misuse or prior diagnosis of a psychological illness, they can be stratified into a higher risk category, which prompt heightened safety surveillance and monitoring. Education can be provided around side effects and safe increases or decreases of the medication. Sometimes, a medication called naloxone, which is commonly known by the brand name Narcan, is also prescribed as a special safeguard. It is a medicine that can reverse the possible ill-effects of opioids and can be given if the patient's family notices any respiratory issues or other concerning symptoms when the patient is taking the opioid medication.

If a patient regularly takes the opioid, their body will naturally develop a physical dependence to it. This means that if taking it for a while, the patient will have a tolerance to the medication. If the opioid was stopped suddenly, the patient might experience unappealing withdrawal symptoms. A way to avoid these is to gradually wean off the medication, as directed by the physician. Dependence is different from addiction, where one may perform harmful behaviors related to the opioid, and there is both mental and physical involvement. I often tell patients, just because they are going on an opioid does not mean they are going to start robbing banks to get the money to get more. I am prescribing it because of a particular physical issue they have as a result of their serious illness, and it is important to see if it helps them live better.

The goal in taking an opioid is to take the lowest dose that has a meaningful effect. Starting with a low (often the lowest possible) dose and increasing slowly is a safe way to get to the target dose. I provide education around possible side effects (most commonly sedation, nausea (both should be temporary), and constipation (which is unfortunately often more of a challenge because a patient is at risk for it as long as they are on opioids).

We talk about the importance of safe dosing, taking the medication as written, and respiratory depression. I create a pain goal with the patient and ask them to keep a log of their symptoms and how many doses they are taking daily. The goal is to keep the patient as active and functional as possible. I am hoping that with the opioid our patient Philip may be able to sleep through the night or get back out into the yard.

Sometimes when a patient is started on an opioid, the family sees the patient become quite sleepy—they may sleep for most of a day! This is often because the patient's pain has been so severe that they have been unable to rest, and now finally they are able to have relief and therefore can catch up on some peaceful sleep. As I will address in the next section, the goal of starting the opioid was not to sedate the patient or get them to sleep awhile—it was for symptom relief. Ethically, the intention here really matters.

In addition to relief of pain and improved functionality, my hope in starting an opioid is that the patient may not need it forever! Often, with effective cancer treatment like surgery, chemotherapy, or radiation, the tumor burden decreases and the patient may not have as much pain. In a situation like this, I would work with the patient to safely wean them off the opioid and get them back to their previously normal life.

WHAT DOES THE CATHOLIC CHURCH SAY ABOUT TAKING PAIN MEDICATIONS LIKE OPIOIDS? DO OPIOIDS HASTEN DEATH?

The Catholic Church supports the use of opioids in a safe and prudent way. The United States Conference of Catholic Bishops has published *Ethical and Religious Directives for Catholic Health Care Services*, which provides moral guidance for any healthcare entity striving to adhere to Catholic teaching.[2] There is a directive specifically on pain (no. 61), which calls for patients to be kept as free from pain as possible, while working to maintain their clearest mental state. As I mentioned in the previous section, pain medications like opioids can cause sedation. It is essential that a safe dose is given and that the intent of the medication is for pain relief, not sedation (which is more a risk at higher doses).

The ethical precept called the "principle of double effect" comes into play here. This principle is worth discussing, as it can be applied to other situations around the end of life (and healthcare in general). The underlying question the principle reflects is: May one perform an action which is intended to achieve a good effect, if it is foreseen that a bad effect will also result? Essentially, the production of a desired good effect that *is* intended occurs along with a concomitant or simultaneous bad effect that is *not* intended. The key lies in the moral goodness or neutrality of the act itself and in the intent.

In the situation of opioids, the goal is pain relief, which is a good thing. Unfortunately, opioids can sometimes cause side effects such as making a patient more sleepy and therefore less able to interact with family. By giving the opioid, the primary intent is only to help with pain, although it is known the patient could get sleepier. It is important to note that the sleepiness is not necessary for the pain to be relieved (the good effect is not produced by means of the bad effect). And the need to relieve pain must be important enough to risk this potential for sedation. If the bad side effect was something much riskier (such as death), the pain relief would not be permitted (the bad must not exceed the good!).

The bishops' directive on pain management applies this principle when it states: "Medicines capable of alleviating or suppressing pain may be given to a dying person, even if this therapy may indirectly shorten the person's life so long as the intent is not to hasten death." The prudent and ethical use of opioid pain medication is for pain or other symptom relief. The intention is not permanent sedation and never is it to hasten death. This can be tough and confusing to navigate, especially in the midst of managing a patient's symptoms. I again encourage honest communication with your medical team (often the hospital care team or hospice) to convey any concerns and help instill peace and confidence that the care is following this principle.

As an additional note, the principle of double effect is applied when a patient may have refractory symptoms other than pain (like shortness of breath, anxiety, or agitation). A medication given to calm and provide relief to a patient may also sedate them, impacting mental clarity. Occasionally, this might be warranted for a time, based on the situation. This should be thoroughly discussed with the healthcare team, the patient, and their family. Providing sedation for sedation's sake (a concept known as "palliative sedation") is something that should be avoided, if possible, as it would prevent the patient from interaction with family and from being able to receive spiritual and emotional care.

WHAT DOES THE CATHOLIC CHURCH SAY ABOUT ARTIFICIAL NUTRITION AND HYDRATION?

The Catholic Church teaches that nutrition and hydration (food and water) by natural means is considered a fundamental right inherent to all humans, not a treatment or medical intervention. Providing food and water to someone is basic, ordinary care. Certain medical situations arise where a person may be unable to take in food and water by mouth, and thus arises the consideration of "artificial" nutrition and hydration. Food and water by artificial mechanism of delivery (most typically a feeding tube) does require a medical intervention for placement. There are different ways to receive food and water artificially. A tube can go into the nose and down the throat to the stomach or intestine (nasogastric, nasoduodenal, or naso-jejunal tubes). A tube can go directly into the stomach or intestine through the abdominal wall (percutaneous endoscopic gastrostomy or jejunostomy tubes). Nutrition can even be put directly into someone's vein through a special IV or port (total parenteral nutrition). When considering these mechanisms of delivery, one can again apply the proportionate versus disproportionate scale mentioned in chapter 3.

As difficult as it may be to think that basic nutrition or hydration could be more burdensome than beneficial, there are situations where a patient may deem it disproportionate to their care. At the end of life, if a patient's body is dying, they naturally may stop eating and drinking. This is physiologically normal and part of the dying process. As the body is shutting down, the body can stop meaningfully assimilating food and water. If a patient has artificial nutrition and hydration, there may be a point where the burdens of continuing that care—such as edema (bodily tissue swelling), aspiration (profound weakness of the swallowing muscles causing fluid to go "down the wrong pipe" into the lungs and cause pneumonia), or shortness of breath (from excess fluid and strain on the heart and lungs)—may be deemed greater than the beneficial effects.

There also may be situations where a patient who is receiving artificial nutrition and hydration gets agitated or delirious near the end of life. Their feeding tube might fall out or the patient may pull it out. Repeatedly replacing a tube for any reason (such as the situation just identified, or when the skin around the tube may have become infected, or when the tube is not working or clogged) can also be quite burdensome.

As outlined earlier, it is always important to think of the "proportionality" of interventions like placing a feeding tube. In certain patient populations, such as those with advanced dementia, many times the ensuing agitation and potential complications of the tube outweigh any meaningful benefit of going through the procedure. If there is a scenario where the artificial nutrition and hydration in the eyes of patient is truly becoming more burdensome than beneficial, it is permissible that it be discontinued. One does not need to feel guilty in this situation or that one is causing the patient to prematurely die.

Many people can tolerate artificial means of receiving food and water just fine, and the benefit certainly outweighs the burden. It is just important to recognize that it is not a "black and white" issue, and there are certain situations, as detailed above, where a patient may deem artificial nutrition and hydration disproportionate (and therefore permissible to discontinue). In general, a person should die from their illness and not because a basic necessity of life like food and water was denied them. Nutrition and hydration by artificial means are meant to help life, not cause more symptoms or an agonizing prolongation of the dying process.

Here are a couple of contrasting patient situations to illustrate this point:

George is a forty-eight-year-old gentleman with esophageal cancer. He was previously healthy and worked as a welder. His oncologist tells him that with treatment he can be cured, but that treatment will be intensive with a combination of chemotherapy and radiation therapy followed by surgery. He has immense pain with swallowing and has lost significant weight since his diagnosis, due to being unable to tolerate much oral intake. Would a feeding tube likely be proportionate?

Helen is an eighty-four-year-old lady with permanent debility from a stroke. She lives in a nursing home and is dependent on others for her care (incontinent of bowel and bladder, needs to be bathed, fed, etc.). Her favorite things are ice cream and watching movies. She has had six hospitalizations in the past year for pneumonias due to aspiration. Speech therapists have tried working with her with no success, as she cannot participate well with therapy and follow their direction due to her limitations. Dietary modification has been attempted. In the hospital, medical care has been challenging because she does not tolerate having an IV in and easily gets agitated, regularly pulling it out and crying out. Would a feeding tube likely be proportionate?

Does artificial nutrition and hydration for one of these patients seem more proportionate than for the other? What good or harm could it do for each patient? You can see again how this process of discernment is quite individualized and most often not black and white.

In hospice care, patients are encouraged to continue living the best life they can and doing things they enjoy like eating and drinking. I know some people consider hospice just for the last days (or hours) of someone's life, but as I explained in chapter 2, hospice is for when a patient desires to shift focus from pursuing disease-directed therapies to symptom management and comfort-focused care. Hospice care can be helpful and appropriate for months, sometimes even years. For some patients, their disease state prevents them from being able to take nutrition and hydration by mouth. They may have a feeding tube that helps them get the nutrition and hydration they need, so they can otherwise live and enjoy their life. I sometimes hear concerns from patients and their families that hospice will not continue the patient's artificial nutrition and hydration once they enroll on services.

Although I cannot comment on the policies that a particular hospice company may follow, medically speaking, if the feeding tube is not deemed burdensome by the patient, there is no reason to discontinue it solely because the patient is on hospice care. As mentioned before, as a patient nears the end of their life, it is natural that their body may no longer be able to adequately assimilate meaningful nutrition and hydration from the feeding tube. They may actually experience swelling or difficulty breathing from the additional fluid, which would worsen their symptom burden. In situations like this it is important that conversations between the patient or their family and the hospice team are regularly had to ensure that the feeding tube continues to be helpful and proportionate to care. If the feeding tube is causing excessive burden or the patient is actively dying and the nutrition and hydration are not being assimilated, it is fine to discontinue the tube feedings. But if the feeding tube is not causing problems and is helping keep the patient comfortable by keeping them nourished and hydrated, by all means it may be continued as part of their basic care.

When considering a transition to hospice for a loved one with a feeding tube, be sure to ask the hospice if continuing it would cause any problem. I recommend doing this prior to signing on to services, to ensure that your values align.

An additional note—it is not ethical to recommend or encourage a patient to voluntarily stop eating and drinking, nor is it ethical for a patient to do so on their own accord. This is the equivalent of a passive suicide attempt and does not respect the dignity of human life. Voluntarily stopping eating and drinking (VSED) is an actual process or "procedure" being employed as a way of hastening death. I have seen it particularly utilized for patients who desire physician-assisted suicide (PAS) but who live where the practice is not legal (more on this in chapter 7) or the patient is ineligible for PAS because they cannot physically consume the suicide drugs themselves (a requirement). For example, some patients with advanced amyotrophic lateral sclerosis (ALS or "Lou Gehrig's disease") have developed severe weakness in their hands, arms, and throat that makes it impossible for them to administer anything to themselves by mouth. Again, a person should die from their illness and not because a basic necessity of life was denied them.

IS IT OKAY TO COME OFF THE VENTILATOR OR STOP DIALYSIS?

It often feels different not starting a medical treatment (withholding) versus stopping one that has already been started (withdrawing). It is emotionally harder to stop a ball rolling once it has already started than just letting it remain still. Yet what I hope to convey here is that they are morally indistinguishable concepts—there is no ethical difference.

In withholding or not starting a treatment, it is determined that the treatment is disproportionate or not something consistent with the patient's goals. In a situation where a treatment may be withdrawn, at some point the treatment was considered proportionate and worthy of a trial. That trial has occurred, and it has not proved beneficial. Although stopping something that has already been started may feel like direct or active hastening of death, it should not be viewed this way. Medical treatments in serious illness, despite their best intent, sometimes cannot fix a situation. Stopping a treatment that is not proving meaningfully beneficial or helping a patient is morally permissible. Viewed in another way, it may actually be unnecessarily prolonging the dying process rather than prolonging life.

This goes back to the concepts of proportionate and disproportionate care and the patient's judgment of benefit and burden. For example, a ventilator helps provide support when the respiratory system has failed. A tube connected to the machine goes in the mouth and down the throat. To help keep it in place, patients are given medications to sedate them, lest they try to pull it out. Patients with a ventilator cannot talk, eat, or get out of bed and have very limited communication abilities (if any). It is not natural for a person to live on a ventilator, and the more days someone is on a ventilator, the more complications they are at risk for, such as developing pneumonia or bedsores from lack of mobility. They also develop profound weakness. From the first day a ventilator is placed, the healthcare team is looking to see when it can safely be removed. After a certain amount of time (typically a few days to a couple of weeks), if this cannot happen, the medical team may start worrying about the tube damaging the patient's vocal cords or other complications. The team may speak with the patient's family about whether the patient would want a longer-term ventilator, something that would require a tracheostomy (where a tube is placed through the front of the neck to support the lungs, rather than through the mouth and throat). This requires a surgery and, if placed, the patient subsequently does not generally need sedation, though they are usually still unable to speak or eat by mouth. The patient may therefore need another small surgery to place a feeding tube into their stomach or intestine for continued nutrition. The hope with getting a tracheostomy is that eventually the ventilator can be weaned off and the patient will recover and be able to breathe on their own. The unfortunate reality, however, is that for many patients complications arise, and patients continue to depend on breathing support long-term.

For many patients it may well be proportional care to go on a ventilator if they need it in the setting of a health crisis. However, if the patient is not showing improvement with the ventilator or is unable to come off the ventilator in a timely fashion, usually, it is not proportional to proceed with the tracheostomy. Therefore, after a trial, the patient's family may elect to remove the tube connected to the ventilator, provide medications that ensure the patient does not experience discomfort, and allow the patient an attempt to breathe naturally without the ventilator, knowing there is a chance the patient may not be able to support themselves adequately and may die. It is important to remember here that the patient is dying from their underlying health situation, not from the ventilator being removed. In those situations, the ventilator was artificially maintaining life, doing its job as a life-support machine. The ventilator was working to help support the patient to give their body time to heal from its underlying health situation. If it seems that the patient is not going to recover from the underlying health situation, they do not need to stay on a ventilator long-term. Again, it is okay to stop something that has become disproportionate to the patient's care. Withdrawing or discontinuing the ventilator is not killing the patient. It is allowing the patient's body to naturally function without the life-support machine.

In the example of dialysis, a patient's kidneys have stopped working (this could be due to a wide variety of reasons). The dialysis machine works as an external kidney, helping to circulate blood and remove waste products from it. It is also a life-support machine. Although some patients start dialysis and can discontinue it later, the majority of patients are on it lon-ger-term (years). Although it definitively impacts their life and routine, they often get used to it and it becomes part of their "new normal." They can continue living life and doing things they enjoy.

There are several scenarios where a patient and their family may consider discontinuing dialysis. Perhaps the patient is nearing the end of their life from other causes (cancer, heart disease, etc.). Perhaps the patient has de-veloped dementia or had a stroke, and dialysis is much more burdensome than before. Perhaps they are experiencing many complications of dialysis (like swelling, blood pressure problems, or skin issues). It may get to a point where the burden outweighs the benefit of the treatment and again, at this point, based on the patient's current or previously expressed wishes, it would be okay to discontinue. If a patient stops dialysis, without that support the patient's body will likely die within a couple of weeks. A med-ical team (often hospice) can help provide education about any symptoms that may arise and have medications available if needed, in addition to other emotional and spiritual support.

The medical situations discussed in this chapter are tough. The process of navigating pain management, artificial nutrition and hydration, and life-sustaining medical interventions can be overwhelming. Decisions for patients like Philip, George, and Helen can and should be individualized to their unique situations. With getting all the necessary information, thoughtful decision-making, and knowing that decisions can be changed over time, I hope you can have more peace working through these chal-lenging issues.

Chapter 5

ADVANCE CARE PLANNING

This chapter will review advance directives and describe how they can be helpful when thinking about healthcare decisions. I will highlight aspects that Catholics in particular should keep in mind when completing advance directives. I will discuss resuscitation options including "do not resuscitate" (DNR) and provide a framework for how to think through these decisions.

MEET MARY

Mary is an eighty-six-year-old lady with a history of high blood pressure who was living independently until several months ago, when she had a debilitating stroke. She was found at home by her daughter Veronica after she did not answer the phone for several hours. Despite being previously independent, the stroke has resulted in Mary having many limitations. Even with good hospital care and subsequent intensive rehabilitation, she continues to be dependent for almost all her care (incontinent, needs to be bathed, fed, etc.). She also has lost some of her mental capacity and is often confused and disoriented. Therefore, Veronica has been helping make medical decisions for her mother, which has been quite stressful. After many discussions with members of the medical team, Veronica made the difficult decision to move Mary into a nursing care facility.

WHAT ARE ADVANCE DIRECTIVES AND WHY DO THEY MATTER?

You or someone you know may have been in a situation like Veronica, helping make medical decisions for a loved one who no longer can speak for themselves. We all hope that we will maintain our ability to speak for ourselves and advocate for our wishes and preferences until the day we die. Unfortunately, for many patients this is not the case. Due to sudden worsening of illness, trauma, or other situations, patients often face big medical decisions when they are confused, on life-support machines and sedated, or otherwise unable to communicate for themselves. It can be very difficult for healthcare professionals and loved ones of the patient to discern what the patient would want in certain circumstances. Advance directive documents can be immensely helpful at times like these.

Advance directives are written documents that help communicate your wishes around your healthcare decisions. They are directions for your future medical care to the people taking care of you medically and for your loved ones. If you have thoughtfully discerned healthcare options and have an opinion, document it! If you are ever in an unfortunate situation where you cannot speak for yourself, any document spelling out your values and preferences will be a major gift to help those advocating for you to have peace that they are respecting your wishes. It is one thing to be able to say, "I know Mom always said . . .," and another to see Mom's wishes directly spelled out on paper. Of course, it is impossible to know in what health scenario you might find yourself and to have specific directions on every detail. But even from basic directives, general values and preferences can be inferred and then further applied to the situation at hand.

Advance directives respect the foundational principle of medical ethics called patient autonomy. Autonomy preserves a patient's self-determination, confirming the inherent dignity of each person. Autonomy imposes a duty on others to respect that worth, as there is harm done when this is violated. It recognizes the right of a patient with decision-making capacity to make decisions about treatments according to their beliefs, cultural and personal values, and life plan, even when these decisions disagree with physician recommendations. A patient can exert their autonomy to not follow medical advice, but it does not extend to the patient the right to demand any and all treatment regardless of benefit or cost.

As a brief aside, to have the capacity to make one's own medical decisions, a patient must meet the following criteria:[1]

1. Communicate a choice that is clear and consistent.
2. Understand the relevant information about their medical condition and the available options adequately to make that choice.
3. Appreciate their situation and any consequences of making that choice.
4. Reason about treatment options, comparing choices and giving reasons for the option they choose.

If patients can do all of the above, they have demonstrated appropriate insight into their situation and are deemed to have capacity for their own medical decision-making.

As a palliative medicine physician, I frequently take care of patients in the hospital who cannot speak for themselves. I can tell you how helpful it is when the patient has previously documented some healthcare preferences! I will review these documents with other doctors and with family members. They provide guidance for decisions concerning the situation at hand.

I also often encourage patients whom I see for palliative care consultations to consider completing advance directives if they do not already have them. Most often, the team social worker is available to help get the forms completed—and notarized, if needed (this depends on state regulations, and different states use somewhat different forms). Advance directives should discuss potential medical decisions that lie ahead, honoring the religious and ethical beliefs of a patient and communicating other values and preferences of the patient regarding their health. Advance directives often include things like naming a healthcare surrogate (medical durable power of attorney), who is someone you would choose to make decisions for you if you could not do so for yourself; completing a living will; and documenting resuscitation preferences. However, not all of these are necessarily helpful or recommended for every patient.

Some advance directive forms may feel like a series of checkboxes, where you can agree or disagree with various options. These generally are not the most useful forms, because they do not allow for the contexts (and often complicated situations) of individual patients. They often do not take into consideration weighing the proportionality (benefit versus burden) of a given option. We do not want advance directives to tie someone to a decision that might accidentally (or intentionally) commit them to refusal of proportionate treatments or commit them to therapeutic obstinacy (doing some treatment or intervention that is truly non-beneficial care). We want advanced care planning documents to avoid statements like "No matter what, I don't want to be connected to a bunch of tubes" or "I don't want any machines breathing for me" or "Do anything and everything to keep me alive." Physicians and other staff should walk patients back from such statements wherever possible because there will be times when the temporary use of tubes or ventilators would be tolerable for patients who have not taken that into consideration when making absolute statements. And there will be times when human dignity demands cessation of medical treatment that is truly non-beneficial (as when a patient's body is shutting down, they are actively dying, and treatments are prolonging the inevitable dying process).

Regarding a medical power of attorney, a patient should choose someone who knows their values, is accessible (easily reached by the healthcare team if needed), and is able to objectively represent the patient's wishes (not limited by emotional involvement). In most states, there is a law providing a hierarchy ordering who someone's "next of kin" would be—that is, the person who could legally make healthcare decisions for a patient. This typically is one's spouse if one is married, followed by adult children, then parents, and so on. It is important to evaluate whether this person would be the best person to follow your wishes and would be able to handle this job emotionally. Sometimes it is most helpful to choose someone outside this hierarchy whom you really trust—and if so, then it is even more important to have this documented.

Consider the patient we were introduced to at the beginning of the chapter. Mary has sustained many health limitations resulting from her stroke that are likely to be permanent. In moving into a nursing care facility, it would be reasonable to see if she has previously completed any advance

ADVANCE CARE PLANNING | 59

directives. Her daughter Veronica brings in a medical durable power of attorney form completed five years ago, where Mary named her husband (deceased as of two years ago) as agent and her daughter Veronica as a secondary (backup) agent. Having this, Veronica can legally make her mother's medical decisions, acting as Mary's voice, representing what she would say, do, and want if she could still fully participate in her care.

Another advance directive called a living will can more specifically highlight your healthcare preferences about treatment options. There is opportunity to share how aggressive you would like your care to be, how you feel about life-supportive machines (both type and duration), and whether you have a preference for a natural death and what you would like that to look like.

Many states have forms specifying preferences around cardiac resuscitation that actually serve as a medical order (depending on the state, these are often abbreviated as POLST, MOST, MOLST, etc.). These are specifically made to communicate the wishes of patients with serious, advanced illnesses to have or to limit medical treatment as they move from one healthcare setting to another (home, hospital, rehabilitation center, nursing care facility, etc.). After completion, these are often signed by a patient or their healthcare representative and their doctor.

Forms like this can be helpful to convey important patient preferences in certain situations, but not everyone needs them. The default in healthcare is to proceed with aggressive medical interventions available (CPR, life-support machines, etc.). So if you are someone that desires this standard (most people are), and no limitations to that standard would be beneficial, then these types of forms are typically unnecessary. The forms are most appropriate in settings where a patient has advanced disease and certain standard care options may be disproportionate to their care.

Considering again the patient Mary, it could be prudent for Veronica to speak with her mother's medical team about her particular situation, and if any of the hoped-for benefits from potential aggressive medical interventions would actually now be lessened. Would her body still recover the same if she went on a ventilator? Or received chest compressions in the setting of a cardiac arrest? Often, after a serious health situation like a debilitating stroke, patients respond differently than they would when they were previously healthy, and it is important to take this into consideration when thinking through these options

AS A CATHOLIC, WHAT IS IMPORTANT TO INCLUDE IN MY ADVANCE DIRECTIVES?

As Catholics, we think of autonomy as embedded within the tradition of stewardship (man has the duty and right to be a good steward of the health and life that has been entrusted to him). We possess freedom, but this freedom is guided by our faith. We also act according to our conscience. The dignity of the person and the preciousness and sanctity of every life should be protected by medicine. The bishops' *Ethical and Religious Directives* states, "The inherent dignity of the human person must be respected and protected regardless of the nature of the person's health problem or social status" (no. 23).

Dr. Peter Morrow, previous president of the Catholic Medical Association, wrote a helpful article on what Catholics should be sure to include in their advance directive, regardless of which form is used.[2] He includes the following:

- The desire to manage and relieve pain in accordance with Catholic teaching
- The importance of assessing interventions as ordinary/proportionate or extraordinary/disproportionate
- The importance of and presumption in favor of providing medically assisted food and water in accord with Catholic teaching
- A clear rejection of prematurely hastening death (physician-assisted suicide or euthanasia) as an end or a means of relieving pain
- The request for Catholic spiritual care, including Anointing of the Sick and Viaticum (the term for Holy Communion given near death, meaning literally "food for the journey")

It is also important to identify a representative to make healthcare decisions as their surrogate in the event that the person loses the capacity to make those decisions. As a Catholic, it is important that this person knows and respects your faith and how that would impact your choices. The bishops' directive 25 states, "Decisions by the designated surrogate should be faithful to Catholic moral principles and to the person's intentions and values, or if the person's intentions are unknown, to the person's best interests. In the event that an advance directive is not executed, those who are in a position to know best the patient's wishes—usually family members and loved ones—should participate in the treatment decisions for the person who has lost the capacity to make health care decisions." Qualities of a good healthcare surrogate include good moral character, the ability to make reasonable decisions under stress, knowledge of the teachings of the Church, and knowing the patient well. They should make decisions in line with what the patient would desire, as long as those desires are ethical.

Some people may not feel they know anyone like this to choose for this role. In this challenging situation, I would suggest detailing as much as you can about your faith beliefs when you document your advance directives to help guide the person making decisions for you. You could also ask at church or talk to your pastor about if there was someone who may be able to help serve in this capacity to help you. Or you could denote in your directives that you would want your pastor or someone at church consulted by your healthcare surrogate when decision-making is happening to help ensure it is in alignment with Church teachings.

Directive 26 states that "free and informed consent requires that the person or the person's surrogate receive all reasonable information about the essential nature of the proposed treatment and its benefits; its risks, side-effects, consequences, and cost; and any reasonable and morally legitimate alternatives, including no treatment at all." This is very important. If you are a healthcare surrogate for someone, it is your duty to ensure that you thoroughly understand the medical situation of the person you are representing, their healthcare options, and the potential issues at stake. Do not worry about taking the time of the medical team or "inconveniencing" them with your questions. You are representing a very vulnerable person who cannot speak for themselves, and it is critical that you do this important job to the very best of your ability.

Returning to our patient Mary, the nursing facility staff asks to sit down with Veronica to learn more about Mary's healthcare preferences. The staff honestly shares their understanding of Mary's health situation and what potential issues may arise in her circumstances. Veronica is able to ask clarifying questions to ensure she fully comprehends everything (questions like those suggested in chapter 3). Veronica also shares how Mary was a generally healthy person before the stroke, how she loves her family, which includes Veronica's sister, Catherine, who lives out of state, and four grandchildren, and that her Catholic faith is important to her. Veronica admits that she and Mary had not had specific conversations about Mary's preferences about healthcare options, but she feels Mary would want to live for her family and would be okay being transferred to the hospital for care if needed.

WHAT IS A "DNR" AND HOW SHOULD I UNDERSTAND AND CHOOSE MY OPTIONS AROUND RESUSCITATION?

DNR stands for "do not resuscitate." This refers to instructions about what medical professionals should do when a person naturally dies (the heart stops and breathing stops). In this setting of a cardiac arrest, the default care is to call a "code" and start aggressive resuscitative measures. Medical staff gets much training on how to effectively and efficiently perform cardiopulmonary resuscitation (CPR), which typically includes chest compressions, intravenous (IV) access, electric shocks to the heart, and securing an airway (often with an endotracheal tube placed down the throat and connected to a ventilator machine). Despite excellent training and evidence-based protocols, CPR still is not always successfully able to "get a person back," to restart their heart and get them breathing again. But it is definitely something that can be attempted.

CPR is more effective the quicker it is started after the patient's heart stops. This is why in-hospital cardiac arrest patients typically fare better than patients who have an arrest at home. With the passing of each precious moment before the heart restarts, there is a higher chance of complications from lack of blood flow to the brain and other organs.

CPR is also more effective for healthier patients with few health issues. A basketball player who goes down on the court with sudden cardiac arrest is likely going to do better than an elderly, frail person with underlying heart disease or cancer.

CPR is tough on the body. CPR in real life is nothing like what is portrayed on television. For chest compressions to be effective, they need to be deep and strong. When done correctly, they often break ribs. If your loved one has a resuscitative effort, you can expect that they will get chest compressions, shocks to the heart, and be placed on a ventilator machine (because when your heart stops, you also stop breathing). Unfortunately, it is difficult to do only some of the resuscitative efforts and not all. It is not like you can go through a list and choose which you want and do not want. It is important to remember that the person has actually died and this is an attempt to try to get them back.

Again, the default for all patients is to have full resuscitative efforts. However, choosing to be DNR status can be something that totally makes sense for a patient and is consistent with their care goals. Some patients who understand the effects of CPR and have underlying serious illness opt for a DNR status in the event of their heart stopping. For them, CPR is disproportionate care. They feel that if, in addition to their underlying medical problems, they then had a cardiac arrest, they would be in a much worse state. For example, think of someone nearing the end of their life from metastatic, incurable cancer. If this happened when their heart stopped, they would like their body to be naturally allowed to die peacefully (without compressions, shocks, etc.).

The honest reality is that for many patients with advanced illness, even if CPR successfully gets their heart to restart, the patient may not be able to be weaned from life-support machines, and this may not be acceptable for how they want to experience their end of life. For other patients, an attempt of CPR and a trial of life-support machines may be completely compatible with their care goals (and still fall within the realm of what they consider to be proportionate care). Choosing resuscitation status is a personal decision and should not be one felt to be coerced.

It is important to note that a patient having a DNR order does not mean that other aspects of their healthcare need to change. The patient can still have an aggressive approach to their health and work to fight illness by way of medical offerings and interventions. A "do not resuscitate order" does not mean "do not treat" or "do not care." Choosing DNR does not mean that you are giving up on your life or not respecting your life's value. It just gives direction in the specific scenario of a cardiac arrest. A patient with a DNR order can (and should) still go to the hospital and be treated for their medical issues. Even issues that need life-support machines (like a ventilator or dialysis) may be proportionate in the eyes of the patient. Like earlier described in chapter 3, each medical decision the patient is facing needs to be weighed and considered in terms of the benefits and burdens it would bring in the patient's individual situation. If something is likely not going to work and very likely to impart significant harm, it is quite possible it could be a disproportionate option.

There are some people who choose to be DNR status and also do not want other life-support machines like a ventilator (in this case they also would have a "do not intubate" or DNI order). And there are some patients that have a DNR, DNI, and also desire their care to be centered around keeping them comfortable and not pursuing other disease-directed interventions (often called "comfort measures" or "comfort-focused care").

Clearly, there is a spectrum of resuscitative status choices. And it can feel confusing! I very much recommend having an honest conversation about this with your healthcare team. It is important to speak about this in the setting of your or your loved one's individual situation. Would different resuscitative measures, in your doctor's opinion, be expected to be successful for you? Would he or she recommend a trial of them? What could you expect your life to look like if resuscitative measures were attempted and worked (or did not work)?

Some people erroneously think that patients receiving palliative care (meaning they have a serious illness) or patients on hospice need to be DNR. Firstly, the purpose of palliative care is to support a patient's care goals, and it is not meant to persuade a patient to be less aggressive or set any limitations to their care plan if that is not consistent with their goals. Often, a palliative care team will have honest conversations with a patient and their family about the reality of their healthcare situation and setting realistic goals, but there is absolutely no mandate what those goals need to be. A patient most certainly can opt for an attempt of CPR in the setting of a cardiac arrest. They do not need to have a DNR status. As described above, the unfortunate reality is that in the setting of serious illness, the chances of CPR being successful are often quite minimal, but this does not mean it cannot be attempted.

A patient's resuscitation status also does not affect their ability to transition to hospice care services, if hospice care is otherwise consistent with the patient's goals. Most—but not all—hospice patients would prefer to die naturally in their home with loved ones present rather than being back in the hospital on life-support machines. A patient does not always need to be DNR status to enroll in hospice. However, it is important to note that most inpatient hospice care centers do require patients admitted there to have a DNR order. Those centers are focused on care of the imminently dying or patients with acute symptom-management needs and are not equipped for aggressive resuscitation efforts. If a patient on hospice desires full resuscitation efforts, they should cancel hospice services and be transferred to an acute care hospital that is more equipped for handling this type of care in the emergency room or intensive care setting. The philosophy of care and the training that inpatient hospice center staffs receive is different than that required to care for a patient who wants more aggressive life-prolonging measures taken.

Returning to our patient Mary, the staff at the nursing facility also asks Veronica how Mary feels about cardiac resuscitation. Veronica again admits that she and her mother had not had any specific conversation about this previously, but she believes that Mary would want a natural death and would not want her life prolonged on life-support machines. If Mary's heart were to stop, given her current debilitated state, Veronica feels Mary would like to have her body be made peaceful rather than receive aggressive chest compressions and shocks, which are likely to not be successful. Veronica signs a DNR form, along with noting DNI with the medical director of the nursing facility.

Chapter 6

UNDERSTANDING THE DYING PROCESS

In this chapter I will describe the signs and symptoms often present when someone is imminently dying. I will work to improve understanding and comfort for anyone who may accompany someone during this time. By reviewing this process, I will highlight specific ways that you can best care and advocate for a loved one nearing the end of their life.[1]

MEET HELEN

Helen is a ninety-four-year-old lady who was diagnosed with Alzheimer's disease more than a decade ago. She has spent her last years in a memory care nursing facility and has progressively weakened and become more debilitated. She is completely dependent on others for her care. She has stopped talking in recent months, becoming completely nonverbal. During a hospitalization earlier this year for agitation related to a urinary tract infection, her three children who serve as her medical surrogates transitioned her to hospice care. Several days ago, Helen became less responsive, began sleeping much more, and started eating and drinking very little. The hospice team alerts her children that she may be nearing the end of her life.

WHAT DOES "NATURAL DEATH" LOOK LIKE?

As Helen's children prepare for their mother's death, they are likely filled with a mix of emotions. The hospice team can be a very helpful resource to guide and support them during this time.

Several years ago, I heard a hospice nurse described as a "midwife for the soul." This really stuck with me. All of us entered the world with a different labor story. How long our mother was in labor with us, what interventions (if any) were needed to assist our birth, what medications (if any) our mother took, who was present at our birth, and whether there were any complications are all aspects commonly recalled and relived. These details are unique to each of our stories and different from those of our siblings and friends. It is the story of how we entered the world.

How we exit the world will also be unique. We can hope for and make a plan for our transition from this world. We can consider what we would like our dying experience to look like: who is there with us, how we look, medical interventions we receive, and so forth. But like birth, a lot of our dying experience is out of our control. You may or may not have had the privilege to witness the dying of another person. Even as a medical professional who frequently takes care of patients approaching the end of their life, I can tell you, the end of life can be difficult to predict. How long the process will take, how someone will look, and whether unexpected issues will arise are often guessed, at best.

A study from the *Journal of the American Medical Association* published in 1999 describes five domains of good end-of-life care: receiving adequate pain and symptom management, avoiding inappropriate prolongation of dying, achieving a sense of control, relieving the burden on others, and strengthening relationships with loved ones.[2] These continue to be used as important standards of care today. Patients and their families should be helped to understand that working to realize these five domains ought to be goals of their end-of-life care and that the patient will be treated with dignity and respect during and after the dying process.

The way the dying process is attended to on hospice is to allow the patient's body to naturally proceed on the course, while monitoring for signs or symptoms of distress and treating those as they come up. Some people are afraid of hospice care services because of a belief that death is hastened. They believe that everyone on hospice services gets a morphine drip, is made sleepy, and then dies. I assure you, this is not the norm that typically happens! Ideally, the patient is cognizant and communicative with loved ones as long as possible—mental clarity is a priority.

As mentioned in chapter 2, if someone enrolls in hospice, a big focus of care is going to be relief of symptom burden. Should the patient become more restless, in pain, anxious, short of breath, or have other symptoms, medications are given. The hospice team members are always surveying for signs of these symptoms, and family members are often given education on how to identify them. If a symptom of discomfort is identified, the principle of double effect described in chapter 4 is invoked here. The lowest effective dose of the medication is given to help relieve the suffering while not intending adverse effects like sedation or delirium (confusion). Some patients will need a bigger dose of a medication than others to find relief, which is due to a variety of reasons. It is a bit of a balancing act sometimes, and it may take a little time to get to the "sweet spot." It is comforting to know that, with hospice, the team is closely monitoring and can check in frequently to make dose adjustments.

Most often, pain and other symptoms can be managed by taking oral pills or concentrated liquid medication under the tongue. Sometimes, particularly when a patient is having more severe pain or is nearing the end of life, they may benefit from a medication by IV. This would ensure that a patient is getting a reliable, regular dose of the medication. It can also be adjusted, based on close monitoring. In these circumstances a patient may receive a drip of a pain medication like morphine. This will not be needed by all patients and is seen more in patients very close to the end of life. Again, the intention is pain relief, not sedation or any sort of hastening of the dying process. However, sedation can sometimes occur as the patient finally gets adequate symptom relief and their body can relax and get some long-needed rest.

AS SOMEONE IS APPROACHING DEATH, WHAT WILL THEY LOOK LIKE?

As patients transition to the end of their life, they often show signs of sleeping more, weakness, decreased interest in their surroundings, decreased oral intake (not eating or drinking as much), confusion, falls, and incontinence. Depending on their underlying diagnosis (cancer, heart disease, kidney disease, etc.), patients may demonstrate additional symptoms, requiring medications for pain, shortness of breath, anxiety, or agitation. Often, a patient may be unable to verbalize these symptoms, and thus it is important to recognize nonverbal signs of distress. By doing a thorough physical exam (particularly evaluating for any skin sores or wounds, rashes, or evidence of urinary retention or constipation) and observing for signs like moaning, a furrowed brow, clenching muscles or contractures of limbs, fast breathing, or a fast heart rate, hospice team members can try medications to see if more evident comfort results. It is not uncommon that doses of medications may need to be increased as the patient nears the end of life. The particular amount of the dose is of less concern than giving a dose that effectively demonstrates improvement in signs of distress. Again, starting low and increasing slowly is the safest way to adjust medications.

Sometimes patients lose the ability to swallow as they near the end of life. In this situation, there are formulations and alternative routes of medications that hospice teams use that can still be effective. Relatedly, some patients will struggle with managing their oral secretions and they will collect at the back of the throat (some call this the "death rattle"). You may hear loud gurgling sounds as they breathe. Typically, when this happens patients are unconscious, not bothered by the noise, and the secretions do not seem to cause them much distress. The sounds are often more distressing to loved ones who hear them. The hospice team can provide medications to help dry up these secretions.

As patients progress toward their death, you may notice skin changes—a purplish color to the limbs is often called "mottling" and can be accompanied by skin temperature changes. Cold, clammy feet and hands, for example, can demonstrate some blood flow changes as the patient's body is shutting down.

Patients also often have a decline in their mental status as they are nearing the final stages of the dying process. This is often accompanied by changes to their breathing pattern, which becomes slower and shallower and irregular. Patients also often have decreased urinary output.

As you can see in Helen, the patient introduced to us at the beginning of the chapter, she seems to have many of the signs of nearing the end of her life. It is critical that the hospice team provide good communication with Helen's family and assess for any questions or concerns during this process. Helping family understand the changes in Helen's body and what potentially to expect can make this time much smoother and calmer for all involved. An attentive hospice team will take time to understand family dynamics and any emotional or spiritual concerns that need to be met.

WHAT IS THE "PERSISTENT VEGETATIVE STATE" AND WHAT DOES THE CATHOLIC CHURCH SAY ABOUT IT?

In some tragic situations, patients will suffer a severe brain injury resulting in an altered sense of consciousness (and severe limitations in their overall functioning), but they do not require life-support machines to live. Although there is hope that patients will arouse and "come out" of this situation to return to a higher level of brain functioning, the reality is that as time progresses, few patients improve. In the particular case of a persistent vegetative state, a patient is awake without being aware. Although often having very limited functional ability, these patients are not nearing the end of life, and their condition can be stable and enduring for years, until the body dies of some independent cause.

These patients, being unable to eat and drink by mouth, receive nutrition and hydration via artificial means. You may recall the news story of Terri Schiavo and the removal of her feeding tube. Pope St. John Paul II stated in 2004 the Church's view that "the administration of water and food, even when provided by artificial means, always represents a *natural means* of preserving life, not a *medical act*. Its use, furthermore, should be considered, in principle, *ordinary and proportionate*, and as such morally obligatory, insofar as and until it is seen to have attained its proper finality, which . . . consists in providing nourishment to the patient and the alleviation of suffering."[3] Therefore, there is a moral obligation to provide artificial nutrition and hydration in this case, similar to others, unless the patient is unable to assimilate it, is actively dying, or otherwise it is clearly disproportionate.

The reality that a patient may not recover from this state is not a sufficient reason to stop it.

Often, when I am speaking with patients about their advance directives, they may share, "I am okay with trying life-support machines, but I do not want to be a 'vegetable.'" I think that kind of remark stems from this concept of the persistent vegetative state, which honestly is quite rare and is a diagnosis where specific neurological criteria must be met. As Catholics respecting the inherent dignity of each human being, the words "vegetative" or "brain-dead" should not be used. In the same address Pope St. John Paul II said, "*A man, even if seriously ill or disabled in the exercise of his highest functions, is and always will be a man,* and he will never become a 'vegetable' or an 'animal'" (no. 3).

Just because someone is unable to participate in life as they had done previously, that does not mean that their life should now be ended, particularly by starvation and dehydration. There is still meaning that this patient can impart to others around them: family, friends, and caregivers. Life still has meaning. If at some point in time the patient developed complications from their condition or directly from the nutrition/hydration such that it was now overly burdensome, it would be okay to consider stopping it, and the patient could pass away peacefully and naturally. But stopping it in this case is very different than stopping it (or not starting it in the first place) so as to hasten death.

HOW DO I ADVOCATE FOR MY LOVED ONE NEARING THEIR END OF LIFE?

Loved ones can advocate by mentioning to the hospice team any observations of distress, physical or otherwise. It can be distressing to witness symptoms of loved ones as they are nearing the end of life—particularly when someone is confused and agitated, combative, or anxious. Sometimes, the distress extends beyond physical symptoms to unresolved psychological, spiritual, or social problems. This is where other members of the hospice team, such as the social worker or chaplain, can be very helpful. They are available to share their expertise—do not hesitate to ask for their involvement.

Witnessing a loved one experience the dying process may well be very uncomfortable. It may even be tempting to ask the hospice team to provide more medication to sedate your loved one, "putting them out of their misery" or expediting the dying process. Remember that relief of suffering is a goal of hospice, but never with the intention or goal of hastening death or killing the sufferer. We must pray for strength and fortitude to accompany the patient along their journey from this life to eternal life. It is not ours to direct or control.

Even if your loved one cannot meaningfully communicate with you during their dying process, it is important that you communicate what you need to them. It is believed that your loved one can still hear you and feel your touch until death is very near. Should you need some time in private, feel free to ask other loved ones or members of the hospice team to give you that. Palliative medicine physician Ira Byock wrote a book called *Dying Well* that encourages good communication with loved ones. If you have not shared with your loved one important messages such as "Please forgive me," "I forgive you," "Thank you," "I love you," or "Good-bye," this may be the time to do it.[4]

Through the course of your loved one's journey on hospice, their treatment plan and goals will be reassessed by the hospice team. It is helpful for you to be a part of these assessments and ensure that your loved one's dignity and preferences are being upheld.

A barrier to some people enrolling in hospice care services in the first place is the belief that all their other medical treatments and medications will stop. I understand the reluctance in this case—this is a very scary prospect! Fortunately, it is not true.

At the time of enrollment in hospice, a patient and their family will review their medical care plan with a member of the hospice team, most often a nurse. Generally, with the transition from disease-directed to comfort-focused care, medical treatments that have been focused on the disease will be discontinued. This includes things like chemotherapy, radiation, dialysis, and blood transfusions, and it is often an okay thing to do because such treatments by this point have either proven ineffective or are overly burdensome (disproportionate to the overall care—see chapter 3). Sometimes there is a treatment that imparts much comfort to the patient, like intermittently having fluid removed from their belly or chest (often present in advance cancers, liver, lung, and heart diseases). In this case, hospice will work to provide a way to continue to drain this fluid, often by placing a small catheter tube that the hospice team can periodically drain in the comfort of the patient's home.

At the time of enrollment the hospice nurse will also review medications with the patient and their family. A general rule of thumb is that, if a medication is helpful in decreasing symptoms or increasing comfort, it is continued—that is the goal of hospice! If the medication does not contribute help in these ways, then there is generally a conversation about the usefulness of the medication moving forward. For many patients with serious illness, they may be on a dozen or more medications. A real issue the patient may experience is something called "pill burden"—the burden of taking so many pills! In many cases, it is a relief to be able to eliminate the less useful medications and pare down the number of pills the patient needs to take daily. Again, with continuation or discontinuation of both medical treatments and medications, conversations should be had between the patient and their family and the hospice team to ensure clarity and comfort with the care.

Particularly in the final days of life, the natural changes of the body make it difficult to assimilate medications, and previously helpful medications may now be unhelpful or even harmful. Bring up any concerns you have with your loved one's hospice team. Good communication will help you have more peace—you never want to be suspicious that the hospice team is stopping helpful medications or treatments in an attempt to save money or hasten the dying process.

Of course, for Catholic patients, advocating for a priest to come visit for Anointing of the Sick should be a big priority. Typically, a patient's faith is noted on their hospice admission, but be clear with the hospice team of this importance. Having a priest come to the bedside, even if the patient is unconscious, can be a beautiful, healing experience for loved ones.

Chapter 7

PREMATURE HASTENING OF DEATH

In this chapter, I will be defining physician-assisted suicide and euthanasia and describing those processes. The Catholic Church's opposition to premature hastening of death and the background for this teaching will be detailed. I will share my conviction that pro-dignity palliative care is the antidote to physician-assisted suicide and euthanasia and how as a Catholic you can practically approach this topic.

MEET MARK

> Mark is a fifty-one-year-old gentleman recently diagnosed with amyotrophic lateral sclerosis (ALS). He is a long-distance runner and works as a highly successful attorney. He has been researching the debility that occurs as ALS progresses and how it may get to a point where he cannot walk, swallow well, or care for himself independently. He does not think that a life like that is acceptable to him, and he has been doing research on his options. He asks for information about physician-assisted suicide.

WHAT EXACTLY ARE PHYSICIAN-ASSISTED SUICIDE (AT TIMES CALLED "MEDICAL AID IN DYING" OR MAID) AND EUTHANASIA?

Physician-assisted suicide (PAS) and euthanasia are both processes where a patient's death is hastened. Although similar, the two are different and the terms should not be used interchangeably.

In PAS a physician writes for a lethal dose of a medication, which the patient takes with the intent of prematurely ending their life. Given its prevalence in media and legality in many states, it is not surprising that our patient Mark would bring this up. As of 2023, PAS is legal in eleven jurisdictions (California, Colorado, District of Columbia, Hawaii, Montana, Maine, New Jersey, New Mexico, Oregon, Vermont, and Washington), and there are active efforts to advance it in additional states. Eligibility varies by state, but typically the patient must be eighteen years of age, have an advanced illness that is terminal, and have an estimated prognosis of six months or less. In some states mandatory psychological screening is required.

Euthanasia (coming from the Greek *eu*, "good," and *thanatos*, "death") notably differs from PAS in that a physician actively administers a lethal agent to a patient with the intention of ending his or her life. While illegal in the United States, it is currently legal in the Netherlands, Belgium, Luxembourg, Spain, New Zealand, Australia, Colombia, and Canada. The Netherlands became the first country to legalize euthanasia in 2002, and laws now extend to those with "unbearable suffering," including children, newborns, and those who have diseases like depression or dementia.

Canada has gained some particular attention because since euthanasia was legalized there in 2016, it has steadily grown in prominence. In 2016, it was legalized for patients with terminal illness. In 2021, it was legalized for patients with disabilities and those with chronic (incurable) illnesses. There have been 44,958 MAID deaths reported in Canada since the introduction of legislation in 2016. In 2022, 13,241 MAID provisions were reported in Canada, accounting for 4.1% of all deaths in Canada; this represents a growth rate of 31.2% over 2021.[1]

WHAT DOES THE CATHOLIC CHURCH SAY ABOUT PHYSICIAN-ASSISTED SUICIDE AND EUTHANASIA?

The *Catechism of the Catholic Church* states that suicide is an act "gravely contrary to the just love of self" (2281) and that voluntarily assisting another in their suicide is "contrary to the moral law" (2282). These acts go against the inherent and inviolable sacredness of life advocated for in St. John Paul II's encyclical *Evangelium Vitae*. The Dicastery for the Doctrine of the Faith's letter *Samaritanus Bonus* declares, "Whatever their physical or psychological condition, human persons always retain their original dignity as created in the image of God" (sec. 3). Someone's life is theirs to give, not theirs to take. Euthanasia is a "crime against human life" and "an intrinsically evil act, in every situation or circumstance" (sec. 5, no. 1). And further,

> "it is a question of the violation of the divine law, an offense against the dignity of the human person, a crime against life, and an attack on humanity." Therefore, euthanasia is an act of homicide that no end can justify and that does not tolerate any form of complicity or active or passive collaboration. Those who approve laws of euthanasia and assisted suicide, therefore, become accomplices of a grave sin that others will execute. They are also guilty of scandal because by such laws they contribute to the distortion of conscience, even among the faithful. (sec. 5, no. 1)

Samaritanus Bonus also addresses the issue of patient autonomy, held in high value in today's world:

> The uninfringeable value of life is a fundamental principle of the natural moral law and an essential foundation of the legal order. Just as we cannot make another person our slave, even if they ask to be, so we cannot directly choose to take the life of another, even if they request it. Therefore, to end the life of a sick person who requests euthanasia is by no means to acknowledge and respect their autonomy, but on the contrary to disavow the value of both their freedom, now under the sway of suffering and illness, and of their life by excluding any further possibility of human relationship, of sensing the meaning of their existence, or of growth in the theological life. Moreover, it is to take the place of God in deciding the moment of death. For this reason, "abortion, euthanasia and willful self-destruction . . . poison human society, but they do more harm to those who practice them than those who suffer from the injury. Moreover, they are a supreme dishonor to the Creator." (sec. 3)

Rather than imparting autonomy and freedom, euthanasia and assisted suicide remove them, taking away any further opportunities to grow.[2]

Let's return now to Mark, the patient we were introduced to at the beginning of this chapter and who is grappling with his new diagnosis.

Patients such as Mark who inquire about hastening their death are some of the most challenging for me as a palliative medicine physician. These conversations make my heart the heaviest as I consider the distress from where an inquiry like this came from. Yet I also have such gratitude for patients' honesty and willingness to talk to me about this. I just wish I lived in a world where it would not even be considered.

My general approach with an inquiry like Mark's is to stop whatever I am doing and make time to be present with him without distractions. He needs to know that I am not abandoning him, particularly in this vulnerable area. He has trusted me enough to bring up this idea, and I want to safeguard this trust.

I need to ensure I express empathy for what he is going through. I show genuine curiosity in the research he has done and commend him on his efforts to educate himself about his disease. I then gently inquire more about his life, getting to know him beyond his disease, to learn his hopes, his values and beliefs, and who in his life is important to him. I ask him what his "best life" looks like, and if that idea for him changes at all in the midst of this diagnosis.

I convey to him that I am hopeful that many of his hopes can still be realized. I share that I am dedicated to walking with him and helping provide the best care and best life possible for him for as long as possible. I explain how palliative care supports patients like him and more about our team model. I share how we exist to help patients like him. I ask whether he will he give me a chance to help him.

If he again brings up PAS or euthanasia, I will honestly share that I feel his life is too valuable to consider this—he has too much worth. He matters to me and to his loved ones. Just knowing him makes my life better. As a physician, I am here to help him live the best life he can for as long as he can. So often, patients have not heard of palliative care and believe PAS or euthanasia to be their only option. I give Mark some time to think about what we discussed and hope to continue caring for him and pray that he will not seek PAS or euthanasia elsewhere.

Mark's initial approach to his diagnosis is not uncommon today, as I described in chapter 2. Yet we know that no disease can rob someone of their worth or value. If someone you know is struggling with their health situation and is contemplating PAS, I encourage you to reassure them of your love, your tireless support, and your desire to know what they are going through. Ensure them of the joy they bring and that they are not a burden. Commit to accompany them on their journey and to work with them to make life the best it can be. Pray for them. Offer to go to a medical appointment with them. Encourage others to also help rally and support this person. Let it be clear how loved and valued they are.

As a palliative care physician, I believe one of my responsibilities is to help the patient discover or rediscover areas of meaning and value that immediate and daunting health concerns may have overshadowed. I do not have an agenda; I work to understand the patient's. I help to restore a patient's sense of their own dignity and encourage them to see that despite significant debility, patients can continue to generate positive activity in their lives and in the lives of others. "The affirmation that the possibility of experiencing, rediscovering, or creating meaning exists . . . even in the last days of life is at the heart of psychiatric, psychosocial, and existential palliative care."[3]

As patients near the end of their life, it is common to desire their end of life to be comfortable, with good symptom management and no pain. They desire mental clarity and the capacity to make their own decisions about their healthcare options. They wish for control of their bodily functions and not to be dependent on others (to not feel like "a burden"). Working through these aims is often what the palliative care team is trying to help people do. Sometimes reaching these aims is not straightforward. Creativity must often be employed, along with good, honest communication, keeping the patient and their concerns in focus.

Some requests for hastening of death come from a place of deep spiritual suffering or existential distress. The patient may feel the disease is a threat to their overall integrity as a person. This can lead to a subjective feeling of loss of meaning in their life, something called medical demoralization. This is critical for the medical team to recognize and address.

IF THE CATHOLIC CHURCH IS OPPOSED TO PHYSICIAN-ASSISTED SUICIDE AND EUTHANASIA, THEN ARE PEOPLE JUST MEANT TO SUFFER?

At the heart of the Christian message, demonstrated throughout salvation history, is God's unfailing love—a love that has no bounds, a love so deep that God sent his only begotten son, Jesus Christ, to become human, suffer, and die for the sins of humanity, in order that we might know freedom from evil and even from death. Through this salvific work, the Christian has hope of eternal life and happiness in the fullness of God's glory.

This victory over sin and death achieved by Christ brings new meaning to every instance of human suffering. In light of salvation, suffering is an opportunity for each Christian to share in this saving love. It was specifically by the Cross that Christ freed humanity from evil and accomplished the work of salvation. In human suffering, we can join our suffering to this same salvific work. Even in the darkness of human suffering, we can love. And it is love that saves us.

The theology of suffering and its meaning for the Christian is deep and complex. There are many books on this subject, and St. John Paul II's letter *Salvifici Doloris* dives into this beautifully and is something I recommend reading if you want to learn more.

The Church does not teach that we are created to suffer through life. It does teach, however, that because of the Incarnation, suffering of any kind has meaning and can even be redemptive in our lives, uniting us to the suffering Christ. We should seek to eradicate suffering while at the same time do the best we can to appreciate its meaning. We should work to decrease physical, emotional, and spiritual pain in our lives, utilizing medical technology and resources available. The fundamental point is that we are free to do all that we possibly can to accompany the suffering and dying person and to alleviate pain within the context of recognizing that human life is a gift and cannot be taken by killing the suffering person themselves.

I view my work in palliative care as a way to help people continue to grow, make meaning, and even flourish during their journey with a serious illness. It is absolutely false that a diagnosis of a terminal illness means life stops. There can be such growth, beauty, and gift of one's life during this journey. With faith, attitude, and support, I daresay this time can be some of the best life one has lived.

A few patients I have cared for come to mind when I think about approaching suffering with a Christian mindset. Their approach is so counter to the typical, it has truly been inspiring to care for them. They seem to embrace the situation they are in and seek to make meaning and good come from it. They view their suffering in light of its more transcendent properties with an inherent redemptive nature. They do not seek suffering, but at the same time they do not shy away from it.

I was recently speaking about palliative care and the Church's teachings to a Catholic parish audience, and a young woman approached me after my presentation. She was in her twenties, admittedly not in the age range of a person who typically has an interest in these topics. She shared her gratitude with me and how timely the talk was for her. She had tears in her eyes as she shared how she was recently diagnosed with multiple sclerosis, an incurable, neurodegenerative disease that will most certainly affect the rest of her life. She honestly expressed that before coming to the talk she felt that physician-assisted suicide was her inevitable future, that this was the only feasible option for someone with her diagnosis. She told me how learning about palliative care gave her renewed hope and that she was so glad to know she had this option.

This encounter was truly touching for me. I was saddened by how little palliative care and the Church's teachings about serious illness and the end of life are known. This young woman was representative to me of how many people are not aware of this and who may fall victim to the cultural push toward hastened death with physician-assisted suicide. And how vulnerable they are! My heart truly goes out to them. I was also struck by the gravity of the message about life-affirming care at the end of life that I believe God has asked me to convey. I was convinced to redouble my efforts to express this truth with love and sincerity, with enthusiasm and renewed vigor, because it is an extremely important message that needs to be shared.

During my time as a physician and attesting to all I have witnessed and experienced, I can tell you that physician-assisted suicide and euthanasia are not abstract theoretical concepts. They are real and they are happening.

Their impact is growing. Our secular culture is becoming alarmingly desensitized. More assisted-suicide legislation is coming in more states, and general knowledge around these practices is limited. I believe with all my heart that the antidote to physician-assisted suicide and euthanasia is the accompaniment of palliative care, which honors the life and dignity of each patient. This is the Catholic response. As *Samaritanus Bonus* declares,

> *Palliative care* is an authentic expression of the human and Christian activity of providing care, the tangible symbol of the compassionate "remaining" at the side of the suffering person. Its goal is "to alleviate suffering in the final stages of illness and at the same time to ensure the patient appropriate human accompaniment" improving quality of life and overall well-being as much as possible and in a dignified manner. (sec. 5, no. 4)

Palliative care's model of addressing suffering from physical, emotional, social, and spiritual aspects really works with the Christian hope and worldview of care for the sick and vulnerable and of their accompaniment. "In times of suffering, the human person should be able to experience a solidarity and a love that takes on the suffering, offering a sense of life that extends beyond death" (sec. 5, no. 4). Palliative care works within the context of modern medicine and technology and provides life-affirming accompaniment. It exists for people with serious illness (and their loved ones). Palliative care is here to communicate that the limitations a patient may have due to their health situation does not impacts their life's value. For each patient is a person willed into being and loved by God, created by God. Each patient is a person to love, not a problem to treat. Palliative care is meant to be that *Good Samaritan*, stopping by the roadside of life to assist a person in need, recognizing their worth.

The last three popes have all specifically supported palliative care. Pope John Paul II stated,

> Palliative care aims, especially in the case of patients with terminal diseases, at alleviating a vast gamut of symptoms

of physical, psychological and mental suffering; hence, it requires the intervention of a team of specialists with medical, psychological and religious qualifications who will work together to support the patient in critical stages.[4]

In his address at the Fifteenth World Day of the Sick, Pope Benedict XVI said,

> The Church wishes to support the incurably and terminally ill by calling for just social policies which can help to eliminate the causes of many diseases and by urging improved care for the dying and those for whom no medical remedy is available. There is a need to promote policies which create conditions where human beings can bear even incurable illnesses and death in a dignified manner. Here it is necessary to stress once again the need for more palliative care centers which provide integral care, offering the sick the human assistance and spiritual accompaniment they need. This is a right belonging to every human being, one which we must all be committed to defend.[5]

Pope Francis spoke to the Pontifical Academy for Life, stating:

> Palliative care is an expression of the properly human attitude of taking care of one another, especially of those who suffer. It bears witness that the human person is always precious, even if marked by age and sickness. . . . I therefore welcome your scientific and cultural efforts to ensure that palliative care can reach all those who need it. I encourage professionals and students to specialize in this type of assistance, which has no less value on account of the fact that it "does not save lives." Palliative care recognizes something equally important: recognizing the value of the person.[6]

Let's get the good word on this beautiful accompaniment out there. There is no time to lose.

IN TODAY'S WORLD, COULD PALLIATIVE CARE AND HOSPICE HASTEN DEATH?

I am deeply saddened and profoundly disturbed to hear of stories people tell me about their experiences of a palliative care team pressuring them or their loved ones to be DNR status or to stop medical treatment, or even worse, stories about hospice "killing" their loved one. Yet it is not infrequent that something like this comes up. In my interactions with patients and from feedback I have received giving talks, it is clear that these experiences are unfortunately much too common. I would like to address that a bit here.

It is a reality that we live in a culture that is becoming more secularized and one that progressively de-emphasizes objective morality. The Catholic worldview is not held by the majority of people and is quite antithetical at times to what is often portrayed in many types of media and by many popular voices. The medical system is not immune to these cultural influences.

I like to compare palliative medicine to the field of obstetrics and gynecology (ob-gyn). With ready access to contraception, sterilization, and abortion being supported by the national academy of the specialty, and with these practices being considered standard options of care, many will say that the field is objectively anti-life and anti-Catholic. However, there are many in the field who do not subscribe to those practices and who practice ob-gyn medicine according to the Catholic faith. Countercultural? Yes. Possible? Definitely. And there is amazing work being done to advance these pro-life practices.

A few years ago, a professional medical society called the American Academy of Hospice and Palliative Medicine came out with a position statement of "studied neutrality" on physician-assisted suicide.[7] You may ask, How can a doctor's organization be *neutral* about the idea of someone ending their own life? Yet, as physician-assisted suicide passes in more states and more people are getting familiarized with it, it is more commonly included in medical education and considered as a viable healthcare option, even as a "standard of care."

I do not share this information to scare you, and I definitely do not want to instill fear that the field of palliative medicine is inherently being practiced immorally. There are so many of us in the field who are honoring and respecting the dignity of life. I share this with you to help empower and encourage you to be the best advocate for yourself or your loved ones. You should take this eyes-wide-open approach with any specialty of medicine you seek guidance from today. And we must safeguard and reclaim the good in medicine and in life-affirming healthcare.

As mentioned in chapter 2, hospice care services are appropriate when a patient is ready to transition to a comfort-focused care approach and no longer pursue disease-directed medical care. I have heard it said that "hospice is giving up." I do not agree. If someone has a serious, incurable illness or has tried an aggressive medical approach to their care that has not given them the hoped-for results, then it is completely reasonable to consider hospice.

When discussing hospice, patients have also told me, "I can't do hospice, Doc, I'm a fighter." My heart goes out to them, as perhaps they have been "fighting" against a terminal diagnosis for some time, despite multiple lines of treatment, hospitalizations, procedures, and progressive debility. I often ask, "What are you fighting for?" And, using their same language, I share that life with hospice care is still a good fight—it is a fight for comfort, for good days with family, for time away from the hospital. It is still fighting; it is just reframing the fight.

Although a patient's life may naturally end sooner by transitioning a fight to comfort-focused care on hospice rather than continuing aggressive disease-directed care to stave off the illness, hospice care should never have the intention of hastening death. As I addressed in chapter 2, hospice workers accompany, witness the dying process, and provide a consoling presence to support the patient and family through that time. A hospice team should be working to optimize the patient's life for as long as the patient has left. This means ensuring they are not in pain, do not have other distressing symptoms, and are as awake and alert as possible, so they can have meaningful interactions with loved ones.

Patients should never be given medications merely for the reason of sedating them or hastening their end of life. I am saddened and disturbed by the stories I hear of people telling me they believe their loved one's hospice team aided in hastening their loved one's death. Sometimes I wonder if there was misunderstanding or poor communication between the family and hospice team. Regardless, if you have any suspicion or concern that the care being provided to you or your loved one is prematurely hastening death in any way, make your concern known! It is far better to fire a hospice team you do not trust than to have something happen to your loved one. There are many hospice company options, and it is important that you feel confident in the care and can trust your team.

Especially if you live in a state where PAS is legal, it is important to speak to the hospice company about their policies and assert your views. After PAS passed in the state where I was previously working, I felt it my obligation to interview the hospice medical directors of agencies with whom I worked. (I did not practice hospice, but was a palliative care doctor in a hospital, regularly referring patients who desired it to hospice care.) I wanted to understand how the hospices were involved with PAS in light of the new law. I learned that the approaches taken by hospice companies were quite varied.

A minority of agencies I spoke with, typically those with a religious affiliation or other association that formerly opposed PAS, would opt out of being involved in the end-of-life care of patients who were PAS-minded, and they would distance themselves from cooperating with caring for patients planning to take their own lives. A much more common approach was to take a "neutral" stance toward PAS by not directly helping to prescribe the suicide drugs or facilitate the process but continuing to care through their end of life for patients who had obtained the drugs elsewhere. The staff of these hospice practices may "assist" with medications for any related symptoms at end of life at or after the time the suicide drugs are consumed. Through my conversations with hospice agencies, it seemed that this may mean providing other medications if the patient is struggling with side effects of the suicide drugs or the drugs are ineffective at ending their life. Then, there were hospice agencies who were open about their more active participation with PAS, with their hospice medical director pursuing the process and prescribing the drugs directly to the hospice patient.

If the hospice agency you are considering will in any way not be respecting your religious views or you feel that there is an agenda toward hastening the end of life, I urge you to look elsewhere for an agency in which the practice of care aligns with your values. Can you imagine your trusted palliative or hospice doctor assisting with killing your vulnerable loved one? The presumption of a therapeutic and trusted physician-patient relationship is severed by such action.

Tragically, this horrific rise of and desensitization to physician-assisted suicide makes many people doubt the acceptability of hospice care for themselves or their loved ones. I get it! But in the midst of this alarming shift in the secular culture, we cannot give up on good hospice care. I want to empower you to be able to advocate for the care you or your loved one deserves that will honor their life, their capacity to love, and their inherent dignity to the very end.

An Added Note on Mental Health

Another added area of complexity around hastening of death comes up when thinking about mental health. Historically, people who are severely depressed or suicidal are cared for medically and watched very closely, even to the extent of committing them to inpatient psychiatric care against their will. The medical specialty of psychiatry is based upon supporting these patients and stabilizing them, saving them from self-harm.

Now, with the rise of PAS and euthanasia, the lines become blurred for these patients. Particularly in countries where euthanasia is legal, the safeguards around patients with mental-health concerns are changing. In some places, a chronic mental illness is an eligible diagnosis for euthanasia. Even losing the "will to live," which can be common with all the stresses of illness, can make someone eligible.

Where palliative care is concerned, I think it is generally a conflict of interest and not ethical for both the palliative care team and psychiatry team to be comanaging a patient's care. What I mean is that if a patient is truly affected by their mental-health issues, these need to be addressed prior to having a reliable and good goals-of-care conversation with a palliative care team. It is not appropriate to discuss one's potential end-of-life options when one is under the throes of an uncontrolled, suboptimally managed mental-health situation.

An example of where this came up for me was when a chronically depressed patient attempted an overdose. She was found by family and resuscitated, and poison control helped the intensive care unit save her life. As the patient also had an early-stage (not as advanced) breast cancer, I was asked to see her for a palliative care consultation. Assuming she had lost the will to live, the medical team asked me to discuss hospice with the patient.

This really bothered me, because patients with early-stage breast cancer often have treatment options with great results. Many times, they can be cured. I judged it to be inappropriate and wrong to be discussing hospice for her breast cancer. It seemed to me that her other problem, her suboptimally managed depression, should be more at the forefront of her care. This was obviously causing her issues, as she had tried to take her own life. This was the issue that needed to be addressed first by psychiatry. The patient needed to have her depression effectively and optimally managed, and only once she was more stable from that perspective should any further palliative discussion be considered.

Palliative care should not be about coercing a vulnerable patient toward electing less care when not justified, or stopping meaningful things. It should never be about hastening death. Physically or mentally vulnerable patients need to be treated with the utmost respect and advocated for—particularly around protection from premature hastening of their death.

Chapter 8

ADVOCACY

In this chapter, I will describe when palliative care services may be helpful. I will share practical ways to bring palliative care up with your doctors and detail what you can expect from a palliative care team being a part of your care. I will also review when the subset of hospice care may be most beneficial. I will share things to look for, particularly as a Catholic, in a palliative care or hospice company, and how to advocate for yourself or your loved ones to ensure getting care that is most respectful of the dignity of life. In addition, I will share about the beautiful graces Catholics can access through the Sacrament of the Anointing of the Sick.

MEET BARBARA

Barbara is a sixty-four-year-old lady with lung and breathing problems. She has smoked two packs of cigarettes a day since high school. Several years ago, she was diagnosed with chronic obstructive pulmonary disease (COPD). At first, she just noticed she was coughing more, and her doctor prescribed her an inhaler. She has had a few "exacerbations" over the years, when she needs to be admitted to the hospital for oxygen support and other medications. In the last year, she started using oxygen at home to help her with breathing. Her doctor has told her that her lungs are now in more severe stages of COPD. It is getting tougher for her to do even minor things, like having a conversation or eating a meal, without significant shortness of breath. She lives alone, but supportive neighbors check in on her with some frequency.

WHEN IS IT APPROPRIATE TO GET PALLIATIVE MEDICINE INVOLVED IN ONE'S HEALTHCARE?

Hearing Barbara's story and how her COPD is affecting her life makes me feel stressed and worried for her. If you have a serious illness like Barbara and you feel you could benefit from more support, I think it is worth considering a palliative care consultation. There are multiple ways to go about this. You can speak to your primary care physician or other physician you trust about your health situation and whether they think palliative care could benefit you. You can learn about it while in the hospital or request a consultation there. You can consult a website such as www.getpalliativecare.org, which has some great resources and a handout that you could share with loved ones and your healthcare team.

Here are some common scenarios where the added layer of support from palliative care may help you and your family:

- You have been recently diagnosed with a serious or life-limiting illness (you have been told you have a limited life expectancy), and you are feeling overwhelmed.
- You have a chronic illness and have been noticing that you are experiencing overall decline in your health. Maybe you have had more admissions to the hospital or you find you just are not able to do what you used to be able to do.
- Your support system or living situation is not what it needs to be, and this is causing significant stress to you.
- Your serious illness is causing you to have symptoms that are debilitating and that affect your daily functioning.
- You find that you are struggling with depression, anxiety, or social isolation related to your serious illness.
- You have upcoming big decisions that need to be made regarding your care direction, and you would like support in these to help feel less overwhelmed and more at peace.

- You are struggling with your healthcare team's approach to your illness, and you feel you are in conflict or on different pages and would like to speak to someone else in healthcare about this.
- You feel lack of meaning or value in your life due to your serious illness and are struggling spiritually with why all this is happening.
- You feel that due to your illness you are nearing the end of life and do not have much time to live and would like support with "getting your affairs in order."
- You keep getting hospitalized for the same things related to your serious illness.

There are also situations where the type of palliative care that may be most beneficial to you is actually hospice care. This may initially come across as shocking or scary, but in reality, if you are expected to qualify for hospice, you may find much more meaningful support and beneficial services. For example, a home-based palliative care team may visit monthly, and you will continue to attend your other health appointments and care, going to the hospital as needed. A home-based hospice team may visit a few times a week and bring all needed medicines and medical care to you so you do not have to get out to appointments or hospitalizations. For many seriously ill patients, it is quite challenging to get up and out of the house for appointments, and it is a true relief to have the care come to their home.

Barbara, the patient we were introduced to at the beginning of the chapter, is experiencing increased symptoms and debility related to her lung disease. It would be very reasonable for her to have a visit with a palliative care team to discuss how things have been going and ways to provide her with more support in her life. Whether it is determined that she would be more helped by palliative care or by hospice services at this time depends on how that conversation goes. She would qualify for either.

WHAT CAN ONE EXPECT FROM PALLIATIVE CARE OR HOSPICE INVOLVEMENT?

Although I wish I could say differently, having worked for years as a hospital-based palliative care doctor, I can attest that our team would most often be consulted in the setting of some sort of crisis. I would often remind my team that although it may be "just another day" of work for us, for our patients and their families it may be one of the worst days of their life. They are now facing a new diagnosis, new limitations to their life, or have learned their prognosis is limited. They are very stressed, and our team is being consulted to help minimize that stress.

So often in the hospital, the healthcare crisis impacts the patient to the extent that they cannot return to their previous living situation. This can be very disappointing to the patient, who prided themselves on independent living and always saw themselves caring for themselves in their own home (or they were the caregiver for another—like a spouse with dementia). Now the patient (and their support system of family and friends) is having to grapple with safe options for the patient to live moving forward. Palliative care can work with the hospital care management team to discuss options. There are many different scenarios out there ranging from independent living facilities to assisted living facilities, skilled nursing facilities, memory care facilities, inpatient rehabilitation facilities, long-term acute care hospitals, and private-duty self-pay caregiver options at home. Unfortunately, palliative care or hospice does not cover these room-and-board type options, but the teams are typically familiar with community resources that are available and can make recommendations for the kind of support the patient may most benefit from.

If palliative care is getting added to your healthcare team or you are transitioning to hospice care, your care will be individualized based on your specific situation and needs. However, I compiled a list of ways you can commonly expect you and your family to be supported:

- You will receive a symptom assessment. Are you having pain related to your serious illness? Nausea? Constipation? Shortness of breath? You may be offered medications (or non-medication lifestyle tips) to help manage these better. Doses should start low and be increased if needed to good effect.
- Community resources that are available will be offered to you and your family. The social worker on the team should perform some sort

of support assessment of your situation and have a good handle on what you or your family would be eligible for. This could include resources on insurance coverage (like applying for Medicaid), housing, caregiver support, food delivery services, day programs, private-duty home support, or safety aides at home.

- You should expect to have a good conversation about the state of your illness, your understanding and preference around your treatment options, and what you most value and are aiming for in your life. This is often called discussing your "goals of care." As a Catholic, this is where you should share about the importance of your faith, how you believe in respect for life to the time of natural death, how regular access to the sacraments is important to you, and so on.

- If you are meeting with palliative care in the hospital, you may learn about clinic (outpatient) or home-based palliative services in your community and receive a referral if appropriate. Should your goals align more with the hospice side of palliative care, you may be able to get a referral for more information.

- You likely will be offered an opportunity to discuss and complete advance directive paperwork like a living will or a Medical Durable Power of Attorney form. You may also have a conversation about your code status preferences and the opportunity to document this in writing, if that is your preference.

- You will have an opportunity to meet with a chaplain, who can provide additional spiritual support to you and your family.

- You will have an opportunity to bring up other stressors that are weighing on your mind related to things like finances, independent living and home support, or how your primary caregiver and more extended family is coping with your illness. Nothing is off the table to bring up!

- Should it be helpful, you can request the palliative care team to assist with clarifying questions you have about your health situation, to advocate for you to other members of your healthcare team, and even to help with creating a mediation meeting with your larger healthcare team to discuss things you are distressed about.

For our patient Barbara, her meeting with the palliative care team should consist of honestly talking about her lung disease, her related health limitations, and what is most important to her in her life. It should include discussing her significant shortness of breath, her social limitations due to it, and her home safety situation (and her support network). It should cover how her hospitalizations have been going and inquire as to whether she feels better when discharged. It should review her preferences around life-support machines, her medical durable power of attorney, and cardiac resuscitation. It should address how she is doing emotionally and spiritually, and if there are other stressors impacting her living her best life. Ultimately, if she does meet criteria to qualify for hospice services, a conversation around the difference between palliative care and hospice would be helpful. This would enable her to determine which program would be more beneficial and preferable at this time (and assuring her she can always change between the two). This conversation would specifically explore the unique features of each and which would be a better fit with her healthcare goals as well as realistically meet those goals.

AS A CATHOLIC, ARE THERE COMMON ASPECTS TO END-OF-LIFE CARE THAT I SHOULD BE VIGILANT ABOUT AND SAFEGUARD AGAINST FOR MYSELF OR MY LOVED ONES?

Unfortunately, as noted in the final section of chapter 7, there are aspects of some palliative care and hospice programs that are most certainly not in alignment with Catholic Church teaching. Although I will be elaborating here on specifics I have noted in the field of palliative medicine and hospice, I encourage you to take an eyes-wide-open approach with any encounter of *any* specialty in healthcare today. For there are also aspects of ob-gyn, pediatrics, geriatrics, and surgery (all specialties, really) where there are opportunities for reverence for life and the dignity of the person to fail to be optimally upheld. I hate that this is the reality of the world we are living in, and it does not mean we should be afraid to receive medical care (or to refuse care you or your loved one would benefit from). It is more about being aware and educated about potential ethical issues that exist and being able to advocate against these and stand up for your values. Any of the following is cause for concern:

- Be aware of misuse and corruption of language by PAS and euthanasia advocates. "Medical Aid in Dying" or "MAID" is how PAS is described by those who support and practice it. "Death with Dignity" is another common tagline of those who support hastening death. "Compassion and Choices" is an organization that works to advance PAS legislation in states (essentially doing for end-of-life issues what Planned Parenthood does for abortion). These terms seek to soften or desensitize what they are doing and to make the concept of suicide more palatable, which is exactly the point. It is important to have awareness and caution with any of these terms.
- Safeguard against hospice involvement in prematurely hastening death. If you have any concern, bring it up with your hospice team, and if you are not getting answers and more peace, get a different hospice agency. As described in the last section of chapter 7, hospice should never have as one of their goals the hastening of a patient's death.
- Be aware of hospice/palliative care involvement in PAS. Unfortunately, particularly in some areas where PAS is legal, there are different degrees of hospice agency involvement with it (see end of chapter 7).
- Look out for Catholic hospitals not following the *Ethical and Religious Directives* (ERDs) from the United States Conference of Catholic Bishops (described further in chapter 4). Unfortunately, just because you are at a Catholic hospital, this does not guarantee that all your care will be consistent with Catholic teaching, since many of the employees, Catholic and non-Catholic, may have not been properly introduced to and trained in the ERDs, or there may not be an institutional culture that is well-formed in the authentic Catholic mission and Church teachings. There are degrees of adherence to Catholic ethical teaching at hospitals, and you cannot make assumptions—you must pay attention and advocate for things if needed.
- Watch out for cooperation of Catholic healthcare entities with agencies not in alignment with the *Ethical and Religious Directives*. You may

be at a Catholic hospital, but you may be referred to a hospice or other care agency that is not Catholic and therefore may not respect your faith preferences. In today's healthcare environment it is common for there to be mergers or other forged relationships between Catholic and non-Catholic entities. You will want to be aware and not assume that your care will adhere to your faith's teachings.

- In palliative care or hospice settings, there may be care "options" brought up to you or your loved one that are not ethically sound and not consistent with Catholic teaching. These may include practices like the voluntary stopping of eating and drinking, overmedicating, or palliative sedation when not indicated, all of which may hasten death.
- Look out for agencies not supporting Church teachings on artificial nutrition and hydration. This is good to bring up in your initial interview of a hospice or palliative care agency (refer back to chapter 4 for further information).
- Palliative care or hospice programs should be well-versed in the available and appropriate advance directive forms. However, I have seen situations where they or others in healthcare (often employees of nursing care facilities or primary care offices) complete the forms incorrectly or imprudently, not erring on the side of the dignity of life or meaningfully beneficial or proportionate care (refer back to chapter 5 for further details).

If our patient Barbara is Catholic, she will want to make sure she brings this up as something important that she values when she has her initial meeting with a palliative care or hospice team. She will want to review any care she may need and ensure that hospice provides those services. This will help her feel peaceful about moving forward, knowing her values will be respected.

AS A CATHOLIC PATIENT, WHAT DO I NEED TO KNOW ABOUT THE SACRAMENT OF THE ANOINTING OF THE SICK?

One of the wedding gifts my husband and I received was a unique kind of crucifix. It was special because it could open up and there was a hidden compartment inside! I was not familiar with the tradition we were being gifted: a sick-call crucifix. Upon further reading I learned that this gift is traditionally given to a couple on their wedding to be hung above their bed. It is ready to be used when a spouse becomes ill or is near death. It is meant to be a reminder to live the wedding vows to be true "in sickness and in health."

Typically, the front slides to unveil the hidden compartment, which contains candles, holy water, and sometimes a white garment. In addition to what it contains, the crucifix can prop itself into the base similar to its position on the altar at Mass. This is meant to be put together when the priest is called, so he can use it when he visits the bedside to administer the Anointing of the Sick. Sometimes the sick-call crucifix can even come with a little bell, to be rung after the priest has heard the sick person's last Confession, to alert family to be able to return to the room. Pretty nifty!

I don't know about you, but growing up Catholic, I was not very familiar with the Sacrament of the Anointing of the Sick. Yet in the course of my work as a palliative doctor, I have learned more about its beauty. It is important to know that as a Catholic you have access to the wonderful graces present in this sacrament. Take advantage of this for yourself or your loved ones! The *Catechism of the Catholic Church* tells us: "By the sacred anointing of the sick and the prayer of the priests the whole Church commends those who are ill to the suffering and glorified Lord, that he may raise them up and save them. And indeed, she exhorts them to contribute to the good of the People of God by freely uniting themselves to the Passion and death of Christ" (1499).

This sacrament is powerful. Until the 1970s it was called Extreme Unction (as it was generally given when someone was nearing the end of life—like in extremis), but the name was changed to reflect the Church's teaching that the sacrament may be conferred on any of the faithful who are in danger of death from their health situation. If, for example, someone is facing a big surgery; if someone has an advanced, chronic illness; if someone is getting older and frailer—these are all appropriate times to be able to receive the Anointing of the Sick. If you or a loved one is in a serious situation, please call a priest and do not miss out on this opportunity for grace—and sooner rather than later!

It is important to know that the sacrament can be received more than once in a person's life. This sacrament can be received as often as needed! The sacrament is instituted by Christ and confers special grace to provide strength. In it, a priest anoints with oil the forehead and hands of the sick person and says the words: "Through this holy anointing may the Lord in his love and mercy help you with the grace of the Holy Spirit. May the Lord who frees you from sin save you and raise you up" (*Catechism*, 1513). Only priests can minister it (not deacons). The sacrament can take place in a home, hospital, or church (it may even take place during a Mass) and can be conferred on one or many persons. If circumstances suggest, it can be preceded by the Sacrament of Penance and followed by the Sacrament of the Eucharist. These three sacraments administered close to the time of death are sometimes called the "Last Rites." If it is near the end of life, this Eucharist is considered the "viaticum" for "passing over" to eternal life. *Viaticum* means "food for the journey" and is true food for any challenges of this time; it is true consolation for the wounds to be endured as the person perseveres in faith and prepares for eternal life. The *Catechism* (1532) also teaches:

> The special grace of the sacrament of the Anointing of the
> Sick has as its effects:
>
> - the uniting of the sick person to the passion of Christ, for his own good and that of the whole Church;
> - the strengthening, peace, and courage to endure in a Christian manner the sufferings of illness or old age;
> - the forgiveness of sins, if the sick person was not able to obtain it through the sacrament of Penance;
> - the restoration of health, if it is conducive to the salvation of his soul;
> - the preparation for passing over to eternal life.

I can attest to the peace that patients and their families find upon receiving this sacrament. Even if a patient has long been distant from the Church, having a priest visit can be an opportunity for deep reconciliation and healing. It is worth considering and bringing up. If you do not have a parish or know of a priest to call, ask the nurse or someone else on the medical team to connect with a chaplain. Regardless of their religion, this person should be able to call a priest, who, if at all possible, should be available to visit promptly.

I have one caveat to note about these sacraments at the end of life in the setting of today's culture where PAS and euthanasia are on the rise. As the document *Samaritanus Bonus* explains the Church teachings: if a person is PAS-minded, they lack the proper disposition to receive these sacraments of healing. A priest who is called to the bedside of a patient who is PAS-minded can visit the patient in the spirit of accompaniment (and there is always hope of conversion of heart), but the priest must show no complicity in the act itself (for example, not being present when the drug cocktail is consumed). This does not imply a non-acceptance of the sick person. With respect to receiving the Sacrament of Penance, "the confessor must be assured of the presence of the true contrition *necessary for the validity of absolution* which consists in 'sorrow of mind and a detestation for sin committed, with the purpose of not sinning for the future'" (sec. 5, no. 11). In the situation of a person intending PAS, "we find ourselves before a person who, whatever their subjective dispositions may be, has decided upon a gravely immoral act and willingly persists in this decision. Such a state involves a manifest absence of the proper disposition for the reception of the Sacraments of Penance, with absolution, and Anointing, with Viaticum. Such a penitent can receive these sacraments only when the minister discerns his or her readiness to take concrete steps that indicate he or she has modified their decision in this regard" (sec. 5, no. 11). Again, there maintains an openness for conversion up to the last moment. For our patient Barbara, if she is Catholic, this can be identified through chaplaincy services, and further conversations can be had about getting a priest to visit and administer these sacraments.

I will close with one last quote from the *Catechism*, as it is such a beautiful part of the richness of the Christian life: "The Anointing of the Sick completes our conformity to the death and Resurrection of Christ, just as Baptism began it. It completes the holy anointings that mark the whole

Christian life: that of Baptism which sealed the new life in us, and that of Confirmation which strengthened us for the combat of this life. This last anointing fortifies the end of our earthly life like a solid rampart for the final struggles before entering the Father's house" (1523).

Chapter 9

PARTICULARLY DIFFICULT TOPICS

This chapter will review some additional issues that arise in the setting of serious illness and at the end of life that continue to be controversially discussed within the Church. I will detail the complexities of these issues, which include brain death, organ donation, and the moral obligation to medically treat.

MEET MICHAEL

Michael is a thirty-eight-year-old obese gentleman who was found lying unconscious on the floor by his brother James, with whom he lives. James had last talked to Michael a couple of hours earlier. Being unable to awaken Michael, James immediately called 911, and paramedics came to their apartment. After several minutes of CPR, paramedics are able to resuscitate him, and Michael is intubated and taken to the hospital. James calls their parents and two other siblings to come meet them at the hospital.

WHAT IS "BRAIN DEATH" AND WHAT DOES THE CATHOLIC CHURCH SAY ABOUT IT?

As we have previously described, medical technology can at times create scenarios that can result in quite perplexing and complicated situations.

For some patients like Michael, life-supportive machines do wonders. Despite having technically died, patients can be successfully resuscitated and after a day or two show signs of meaningful brain function (acting independently, following commands). They are able to be weaned off the machines and are truly given a second chance at life.

Other patients are not always so fortunate. Despite all aggressive interventions and attempts of life support, there do not seem to be signs of organ recovery. The lungs, heart, kidneys, and liver can all be failing, and other complications such as infections can also arise. Most importantly, though, there may be no signs of brain recovery. The patient may not have reflexes, and their brain may not even be able to tell their body how to breathe (brain and brainstem failure). This is a very tough situation, where the medical team may make a determination of "brain death."

Truly meeting criteria for brain death is complex and remains a controversial topic within Catholic medical ethics. If brain death is being considered, the process and the criteria should be well-explained to family or other healthcare surrogates along the way; it should not come as a shock to them. Any consideration of organ donation should be delayed until after this process has been completed. (There must always be medical determination of death—brain death or otherwise—prior to organ donation).

SHOULD I BE AN ORGAN DONOR?

The *Catechism of the Catholic Church* states the following about organ donation:

> Organ transplants are in conformity with the moral law if the physical and psychological dangers and risks incurred by the donor are proportionate to the good sought for the recipient. Donation of organs after death is a noble and meritorious act and is to be encouraged as a manifestation of generous solidarity. It is not morally acceptable if the donor or those who legitimately speak for him have not given their explicit consent. It is furthermore morally inad-

missible directly to bring about the disabling mutilation or death of a human being, even in order to delay the death of other persons. (2296)

And the *Ethical and Religious Directives* declares,

The transplantation of organs from living donors is morally permissible when such a donation will not sacrifice or seriously impair any essential bodily function and the anticipated benefit to the recipient is proportionate to the harm done to the donor. Furthermore, the freedom of the prospective donor must be respected, and economic advantages should not accrue to the donor. (30)

Let us now break this down a bit. The gift of life through organ donation is inherently a selfless and wonderful thing. The Catholic Church is not opposed to this. The technological progress that has made this possible has saved countless lives. I spent time during medical school rotating on the surgery transplant service, and it was exciting and beautiful to see patients getting a new lease on life through the transplantation of an organ. The process can also give organ donors an opportunity to provide a truly charitable, selfless act and permit their bereaved families to see some tangible good come from their dying. In thinking about organ donation through the lens of the Catholic faith, the "respect for life, human dignity, bodily integrity, and the desire to relieve suffering should guide transplantation care."[1]

The tricky thing that sometimes arises (and what Church teaching cautions to safeguard against) is that care around a donated organ (or its recipient) can supersede care of the person whose organ it originally was (the donor). It is clear that the recipient of the potentially donated organ is not more important than the donor, and the lives of both must be equally respected. In the case of the donor, the harm and risks of the donation and transplantation of their organ must be proportionate to the good done to the organ recipient. The benefits to the recipient must outweigh the burdens to the donor.

Never should there be coercion to get someone to donate their organs. Never should someone be compensated financially in donating an organ. Never should organs be donated without explicit informed consent of the patient or their healthcare surrogates. Never should someone's death be hastened so as to pursue the transplant of their organs to delay the death of another.

Organ donation is not obligatory and is something that can be decided near the time of your death by you or, if you are no longer able to make decisions for yourself, by your designated healthcare surrogate (who you trust would be following your wishes and respecting your values). In my experience, and in thinking through Catholic teaching on this, while there are different approaches, it has been my experience with patients that it is better to defer your decision to be an organ donor to your loved ones if you are found in a situation where this issue would come up (and by all means, share with them your preferences around this ahead of time). What I mean is, it is better to wait than saying yes to being an organ donor at the Division of Motor Vehicles (DMV) office, when you do not yet know or understand the context of the health situation you could find yourself in. This is similar to not completing advance directive forms in a way that could "lock" you in to healthcare choices that are not consistent with respecting your life or values. It is important that you or your healthcare surrogate can have an opportunity to have an explicit informed-consent conversation about this with members of your healthcare team in the context of your particular healthcare situation.

In some states, an organ procurement organization (OPO, a federally affiliated, not-for-profit organization responsible for recovering organs from deceased donors for transplantation) with proof of a patient's assent to be an organ donor on their driver's license can trump family surrogates' decisions.[2] This is important to think about as, although we cannot predict the health situation we may find ourselves, I know I would like the context of the situation I am in to be taken into consideration with making big medical decisions (like potentially donating my organs). Because of these circumstances, rather than at the DMV, I feel the appropriate place for an informed discussion on the option of organ donation is at or near the bedside of the patient, with the patient's healthcare surrogates or family present, as well as members of the medical team (ideally including palliative care if available) who can provide unbiased education, insight, and information about the patient's prognosis. If, after this, the healthcare surrogates decide to learn more about organ donation, then they can meet with the OPO. There should be a hospital policy in place on how the OPO should be contacted (typically by nursing). Through all this, it is important to remember that there is no moral obligation to donate organs; it is only an option if the moral conditions are met.

In my time working with organ transplantation in medical school, I also saw situations where a family member or friend would give the gift of their organ voluntarily to a loved one in need. This is typically seen in the case of renal failure and kidney donation. As the donor has two healthy kidneys and can continue normal living with just one, they consider donating one. This is an extraordinarily generous gift and again is something that must be evaluated seriously to determine that it is proportionate (not causing too great a harm to the donor and at the same time providing substantial benefit to the recipient), that there is good informed consent, that it is an act free from any coercion, and that this serious need of the recipient cannot be fulfilled in any other way.

In thinking about our patient Michael and organ donation, first a healthcare surrogate should be determined, and the healthcare team should work to understand more of who Michael is as a person and his values and preferences around his health. The team should also work to communicate with Michael's surrogate all that is understood about his current health situation and prognosis. If the prognosis is such that Michael is not going to survive this illness and he is a potential organ donor, then the topic should be broached with family. Family can have an opportunity to ask any questions of the team and can then decide how to proceed.

AS A CATHOLIC, ARE THERE SOME MEDICAL TREATMENTS THAT ARE OBLIGATORY?

From the *Ethical and Religious Directives*: "While every person is obliged to use ordinary means to preserve his or her health, no person should be obliged to submit to a health care procedure that the person has judged, with a free and informed conscience, not to provide a reasonable hope of benefit without imposing excessive risks and burdens on the patient or excessive expense to family or community" (32).

Again, as a Catholic there is a duty to protect life, but not one to preserve it at all costs. If something is proportional to their care, a patient should pursue it. But if they deem it disproportionate, they are not bound to. How this is interpreted can look different for different patients and can present in quite challenging ways.

I recall a patient that came into the hospital with shortness of breath and was found to have a very dysfunctional heart valve. The cardiology team met with her and gave her the good news that her bad valve could easily be replaced with a procedure to put in an artificial valve. However, the patient was adamantly opposed to this, surprising the cardiology team, who felt this procedure was low-risk and that if she did not get it, she would most certainly die in a few weeks or months. Frustrated at her insistence on forgoing the procedure, they consulted palliative care (me) to further understand the situation.

When I met the patient, she was accompanied by several family members. I learned that she was in her eighties and was fiercely independent, having been widowed several years earlier. Her family shared that she was the anchor in the family and had raised many of the grandchildren in addition to her children. She was not someone who went to the doctor or liked to take medication. She prioritized staying active, and this in her mind kept her healthy.

In the consultation, I assessed her understanding of her heart condition and the care options in front of her. She clearly was able to appreciate the risks and benefits of the valve replacement and consistently stated she did not want it. She was not interested in any kind of procedure or surgical intervention to her body. We discussed that, without it, she would likely continue to have symptoms, like the shortness of breath, which would further worsen. She would come to a place where she would be unable to be as active and, ultimately, she would die from this. I tried to convey accurately to her what the procedure would be like (there are some great videos on YouTube!) and even drew some pictures. It was difficult to pinpoint exactly why she was opposed to the procedure (I considered things like financial reasons, personal spiritual beliefs, experiences of a loved one with a like procedure, etc.), but it was clear it was not something she felt was manageable. Finally, I shared that if she did not get the procedure, I would recommend hospice care to help with any issues that might arise. She and family agreed to this, and she was discharged from the hospital and home on hospice a day or two later.

This was a difficult consultation for me as, in my view, the procedure did not seem excessively burdensome and would give great benefit; therefore, it was proportionate to her care and should be pursued. However, if in the eyes of the patient (with capacity to make their own medical decisions) it is not, I have to respect their choices. This issue, though somewhat rare, does come up from time to time and can be extremely frustrating to witness. To see a family member, friend, or patient not pursue (or even attempt) a treatment that you feel could help them can be truly difficult to understand. Yet, if there is an informed conversation with a patient who understands their options (and has full capacity to do so—meaning they are not confused, demented, or suffering from another mental condition where they are not fully able to advocate for themselves; i.e., they are not depressed, manic, psychotic, or suicidal)—their decision, as difficult as it is, should be respected.

For our patient Michael, there may come a point where the healthcare team does not see his condition improving and there arises the dilemma of when to stop disease-directed treatment and transition to comfort-focused care. At times, the reality of life-supportive technology transitions more from sustaining one's life to prolonging one's death. There may come a point where it is recommended to stop the life-supportive technology and let his body die on its own. There may be a situation where a given treatment may be truly considered "non-beneficial." I prefer this term over "futile," as it is difficult to truly determine whether something is objectively futile (a good definition of futility is "a medical intervention's inability to deliver the benefit for which it is designed"[3]). With medical technology today, it honestly seems there is always something more that can be done or tried. But just because it can be tried does not always mean it *should* be tried. The question to be asked is: Does the intervention increase the likelihood of reaching the patient's goals, with acceptable related burden?

It is completely permissible to have limits on your or your loved one's care. This is one of the reasons advance directive conversations and forms are so important and helpful. If your or your loved one's medical team communicates that a specific treatment is not considered to be very beneficial and does not recommend it, it is important that you ask any questions you have so that you fully understand their reasoning. Although you may hate the situation you or your loved one is in and want things to be different, it is important that you feel at peace with the plan of care. If after communicating you truly do not feel at peace with not offering or discontinuing a certain treatment, you may inquire about the feasibility of a time-limited trial to see if the treatment may be able to be given for a finite amount of time to see if it provides any hoped-for effect. This is also likely a good time to inquire about having a palliative care team be involved in the care if possible.

Chapter 10

PORTRAIT OF A PALLIATIVE MEDICINE PHYSICIAN

In this chapter, I will share how I define my role as a palliative medicine physician and the unique aspects the palliative team adds to patient care. I also want to share with you how my faith beliefs are incorporated into the work.

MEET ANDREW

Andrew is a seventy-five-year-old gentleman, previously healthy, who has recently been diagnosed with congestive heart failure (CHF), an incurable condition. He has shortness of breath and some swelling in his legs and recently has not been able to go golfing like he used to. He is hospitalized to work at improving his symptoms, and his medical team consults the palliative care team because since receiving his diagnosis, Andrew is not eating, will not work with physical and occupational therapy, and has been withdrawn, sitting in his hospital room with the lights off and a washcloth over his head. His family is distraught to see him like this when he is usually energetic and upbeat. His doctors and nurse ask the palliative team to talk to him about hospice care.

WHO AM I AS A CATHOLIC PALLIATIVE CARE PHYSICIAN?

You may know someone like Andrew, someone whose life is completely turned upside-down by a new diagnosis. As a palliative care physician, hearing about Andrew makes me want to jump up and try to help. As I have touched on earlier in this book, palliative care, hospice, and my role as a physician practicing this kind of medicine are often misunderstood. Add the fact that I am trying to live and practice according to Catholic Church teachings, and people struggle with trying to fit me into a specific "box." For me personally, the way I practice palliative care is motivated by my faith. When I describe who I am and what I believe it means to be a Catholic palliative care physician, I use four foundational descriptions: *advocate, guide, counselor,* and *cheerleader.* I will briefly elaborate on each here, and hopefully this will help shed some light on how my work plays out—and why I view it as a special ministry.

ADVOCATE

As a palliative care physician, I have the privilege of time to get to know who a patient is beyond their diagnosis. It is my job to work to understand a patient's beliefs, values, and healthcare preferences, so I can help recommend value-concordant care and represent the patient well to others on their medical team. I do this by listening and then advocating.

The patients for whom I care are often in the midst of serious illness or nearing the end of life. They often have limitations that make them quite vulnerable. Part of my job is to advocate for them in light of these vulnerabilities. Can the patient adequately understand their medical situation? Do they need hearing aids, glasses, dentures, or an interpreter to help them communicate more effectively? Are there basic things that hospital staff and family can do to help improve confusion (delirium) in the hospital (things environmentally like turning on the lights and opening the blinds during the day, as well as orientation questions like reminding the patient of the date and where and why they are at the hospital)? Do they need a healthcare surrogate? I work to dig deeper below the surface to help others on the medical team recognize any barriers to care and how these can be rectified. If I do not bring these important barriers to light, who will? It is my role to ensure respect for the patient's inherent dignity, regardless of their limitations.

Sometimes, in advocating for patients, I feel a bit like a bulldog. The way I staunchly represent who the patient is and what they need can be unpopular among other hospital staff. It can mean things that take more time or add steps to care. Yet I am dedicated to serving the needs of patients and to fearlessly standing up for their faith beliefs, rectifying limitations in care, and holding up standards of medical care excellence. I try to live by the belief that each patient is a person to care for and love, not a problem to treat.

I want to will the patient's good. I "go to bat" for them. Sometimes I almost feel like a defense attorney, someone in their corner, representing them. A physician friend of mine described this "defense attorney" role that a good physician takes. He described how physician-assisted suicide (PAS) or euthanasia is so antithetical to this role. For if as a physician, you begin the PAS process with a patient, you are no longer the defense attorney but have switched to the side of the prosecution. And if you are going through the eligibility criteria for PAS, you become the patient's judge, someone even more removed from the patient's side. And if you actually "succeed" in obtaining the drugs to prematurely end the patient's life, you become their executioner. This is so distant from the defense attorney role and so incompatible with who I am as a Catholic palliative doctor, desiring and advocating for my patients' flourishing to the end of their natural life.

GUIDE

People who know me know that hiking is one of my favorite pastimes. When I moved out west for my medical training, I told myself that on any day off work, I needed to do what I could to get out on the local mountain trails. I just love following a trail, discovering the beauty of nature, and often finishing by reaching the goal of a beautiful vista or majestic peak.

Navigating the healthcare system is rough and overwhelming. Many times patients do not adequately understand their medical problems, their care options, and the consequences of those different options. As a palliative care physician, I help patients and families proceed through the murkiness, shedding light on the path forward. I ensure they have the correct understanding and take the time to answer their questions and get them the answers they need. I do everything I can to help provide meaningful health education to the patient and their family. If there are major gaps,

I help communicate these to the rest of the patient's medical team, to get everyone on the same page.

In palliative care training, we receive special training in communication. We learn how to combine empathy with honesty and to have the courage to truthfully communicate even when the news we have is not good. Shedding light on a patient's path means empowering them with knowledge so that they are better and more peacefully able to make decisions. As a physician, I believe this is something we are obligated to do. As difficult as discussing a certain issue with a patient and family may be, gently, tactfully, and truthfully providing information can be really freeing to the patient and a true gift to guide them how to best live the best life possible.

COUNSELOR

I like to think of palliative care as providing a humanizing touch. Our team has the ability to sit and connect with people. When I enter a patient room, I try to remove all distractions. I verify with the patient, family, bedside nurse, and other team members that it is a good time to visit. I place a sign on the door that states that a palliative care meeting is in progress and to please not disturb. If there is not a spare chair in the room, I bring one in. I view the hospital room like the patient's living room at home—I am entering into their private, personal space, and I want to give the patient as much control as possible when often they have been stripped of much of this by being in the hospital.

I often tell patients that I am there to provide support to them and everyone who loves them. There is no aspect of stress related to a serious illness that is out of our scope to talk about. I am here to help provide communication (however difficult), creative family and patient support, and symptom management. A common phrase in palliative care is that we help patients "hope for the best, while preparing for the worst."

The patient's loved ones often feel quite powerless when their loved one is sick in the hospital from a serious illness. They want to help but do not quite know how. One thing that has been helpful in my practice is to provide them with some "homework." I give them a paper that is blank other than the outline of a picture frame. Its instructions are to provide a photo that represents who the patient is and how they would like their healthcare team to see them. Where I have worked, this has been very positively received, and not only does the family bring in a photo, but often they bring in a whole posterboard or photo collage! I recall one family of a patient unconscious on a ventilator machine bringing in a photo of the patient on his riding lawn-mower, with his poodle on his lap and holding a beer in his hand. It was so illustrative of who this patient was and helped the whole medical team better connect with him as we fought to get him through his acute illness.

Particularly during the COVID-19 pandemic, our palliative care team worked to provide a humane and personal touch. It was devastating that patients could not have visitors or even had to face the prospect of dying alone. There was much stigma around the disease, how a patient contracted it, and their vaccination status. For patients in isolation, our team worked to provide meaningful connections for them with the outside world. Whether this was through photos and letters from loved ones, or arranging window or virtual visits, we worked to humanize their situation as best we could.

I really appreciate that I get to use my creative side when counseling patients and their families. I ascertain how patients best receive and understand information. Sometimes I draw pictures or find videos to help explain their medical situation. I may bring additional articles that help shed light on the situation. At times, it is like a puzzle trying to figure out how to help a patient realize their goals (or to help unlock some obstacle or misperception that is a barrier to care or causing conflict or distress), and I am up to the challenge!

CHEERLEADER

This may be one of my favorite roles in being a palliative care physician. Although I can be rather peppy and spirited at times, I was not a cheerleader in real life. However, I really enjoy encouraging others and "pumping them up." What unfortunately can happen in the hospital is that a patient may be diagnosed with something and subsequently feel that their life is no longer worth living. They may feel so overwhelmed that they feel their very existence would be a significant burden to their loved ones and to the world. They may feel they do not want to consider any treatment options. They may stop working with the care team in the hospital, preferring to withdraw. In extreme cases, they may inquire about prematurely hastening death with physician-assisted suicide.

In the majority of these situations, patients are experiencing real medical demoralization. The core of their perceived identity has been shaken by a diagnosis or other health news. They feel disintegrated. Well, I am not going to give up on these people. It is my job to remind them how their life is not defined by this and to help reinstate their hope. At times, this has meant bringing back some joy into their lives in a tangible way. I recall the time a lady was in the hospital for weeks for the complications of abdominal surgeries. Intermittently, she just wanted to give up. I learned that prior to her first surgery she had loved to travel, and she had shared with me about a particular meaningful trip to Egypt. Well, our team "took" her to Egypt—complete with a sphinx headdress, photos of the pyramids, and staff members joining us to parade into her room to "walk like an Egyptian." She started dancing with us! It was beautiful to see.

Another patient learned he was going to have his right leg amputated after his left leg already had been. This was devastating, and he was feeling very low. It also meant he could not take his anniversary trip to the Bahamas with his wife the next month. So, our team brought the Bahamas to them and turned his hospital room into the tropics.

Not only do these situations bring joy to the patients, but the joy spills over to hospital staff as well. You may be familiar with the film *Patch Adams*, starring Robin Williams. A true story depicting a medical student who wants to connect with patients beyond their diagnoses, it touches on a lot of aspects of palliative care. There is one memorable scene where a hospitalized elderly lady shares her dream of always wanting to swim in a pool full of noodles. Patch Adams actually creates this for her and swims around in it with her! Although I have never had this request, I do often think when I care for certain patients, "What is their swimming pool full of noodles?"

And so, let us now return to Andrew, the patient we were introduced to at the opening of this chapter who is struggling with a new diagnosis of heart failure and some symptoms related to it and is grappling with what this means for his life.

I was asked to see him as his response to his new diagnosis seemed to be one of giving up on life, and his medical team thought perhaps the best path forward was hospice. Well, my team went in and the first thing we did after introducing ourselves to him and his family was to open the blinds and turn on the lights. I sat by Andrew's bedside, and we talked about his health situation. He shared how he felt the heart failure was a death sentence. He had friends who had died of heart troubles. Life to him now was not worth living. I educated him and his family about CHF and symptom management. I told him about home palliative care. I told him that he could still expect good days and good things despite this diagnosis. That he still had things to do. That, just by meeting him, he made my life and the lives of my teammates better. (By the way, he did not have advanced CHF and would not even have met hospice criteria.)

The next day I headed to his room when the medical team's morning rounds were just finishing. They gave a little cheer, and the attending physician gave me a high five. I peered into the room. The lights were on, and Andrew was up, eating, joking. The family members came to me, one of them crying, and said, "You brought him back to us, Doc, thank you. We now have hope."

I am not going to give up on people! My Catholic faith forms who I am as a palliative care physician. How I see and respect the dignity of the vulnerable, my love and desire to will the good for the other (and to remember that this is a person willed into being and loved by God, created in God's image and likeness), my desire to practice virtuous medicine, and my goal to operate by the highest ethical standards—all are rooted in the Catholic faith.

It is truly a gift and a privilege to have this professional vocation and do the work that I do. To accompany people in moments of crisis, in intense suffering and vulnerability, provides such an opportunity to provide meaningful support. I may not be able to cure or fix a patient, but I can work my very hardest to creatively reduce suffering and to help people continue to grow, to live, and, I daresay, even to flourish, despite serious illness.

I compare being a Catholic palliative care doctor to being a Catholic obstetrician, as these specialties are devoted to caring for the "bookends" of life. We are tasked with supporting, promoting, and protecting dignity at these vulnerable times of life, when patients are at risk of being undervalued, undermined, and exploited. We both fight abortion. In palliative care, we are counteracting abortion at the end of life.

Good palliative and end-of-life care is a pro-life and pro-dignity issue. At the same time it is also a social-justice issue—to accompany the sick and dying. People deserve to have access to appropriate symptom management, emotional and spiritual support, and to receive the respect of a good, natural death. I believe access to good palliative care is a human-rights issue, and it's definitely a Catholic issue. The *Catechism of the Catholic Church* says, "Palliative care is a special form of disinterested charity. As such it should be encouraged" (2279). Palliative care elevates the humanity of the person and emphasizes their intrinsic dignity.

There are times I have cared for a patient and their family and someone says, "No one has ever cared for me like this before." Or there is a patient deemed "difficult" by hospital staff and I am included in a meeting to help devise a solution to a conflict. In the meeting I take the time to focus on the dignity of the patient, however difficult. Multiple staff members will later come up to me and say, "I want someone like you caring for me if I am in the hospital or nearing the end of life." I am touched by the kindness of these remarks, but also saddened. What I do should not be out of the ordinary, but unfortunately the reality in healthcare is that, for a myriad of reasons, too often we are desensitized to patient suffering, become low in empathy, and even forget the humanity of the patient right before us.

And, despite my best attempts, I do not practice my ideal of palliative medicine perfectly. I am not immune from the human struggles of grappling with witnessing suffering, injustice, and other difficult situations. It can feel very discouraging at times, and people often ask how I can stay joyful and not "bring it all home" at the end of the day. I think it is my faith that helps me keep things in perspective, as well as a deep trust in God's mercy and goodness that extend far beyond my understanding. A wise friend early in my career encouraged me at the end of each day to "hang up the proverbial stethoscope" and leave work at work. It also helps to have a supportive palliative team with which to debrief and share challenges. None of us are meant to experiences life's challenges alone!

I just tell myself: I must not become discouraged. I recognize that threats against human dignity are abundant. More states are legalizing PAS. Yet, as a Catholic, I am part of a Church that stands for beauty, goodness, and truth. I can work each day to sanctify myself and the world around me through my work and the way I care for patients and their families. I can choose each day to see each patient as a person to love rather than a problem to treat. I can radically love these patients in the midst of this world and bring our Church teachings to life in the trenches of healthcare. And if one day I fall short, the next day I begin again, grateful for God's mercy and prayerfully maintaining hope through faith in him. This is what I believe to be authentically Catholic palliative care.

WHAT IS A GOOD DEATH?

In his book *The Anticipatory Corpse: Medicine, Power, and the Care of the Dying,* Jeffrey P. Bishop writes about a person facing cancer: "Death threatened to take it all away, yet death also put the whole of her life into perspective."[1] I personally can attest how death does this. Taking care of patients facing this experience has done this for me. Starting my palliative care fellowship, I remember how food tasted better, colors appeared brighter, and music sounded sweeter. My senses were literally heightened as I more deeply realized life's preciousness and lack of permanence. Although my personal mortality was not being immediately threatened, being around death and thinking about mortality changed how I approached life. Acknowledging death, that there is a finite end to the mortal life, and that medicine cannot fix everything helped me accept a new philosophy of practicing medicine. Instead of working to cure or ameliorate, as I had been taught in medical school and been trained in internal medicine residency, as a palliative medicine physician I now had to learn how to "be with" suffering and to work to creatively improve patients' quality of life, in whatever way it might be threatened or compromised.

As a palliative medicine physician, I have learned how to be more comfortable around suffering. Sometimes what patients need most is an emotional, empathic response to their concerns, rather than a cognitive, solution-based answer. In my work, I have seen such a variety of responses to suffering. I have had the privilege to witness a large number of deaths, many—though not all—of which I would classify as "good deaths." Although it may sound a bit morbid, a few years ago I performed the exercise of writing my own epitaph and thought about what I hoped for in my own departure from this world. When I consider what is a good death, the following characteristics come to mind:

1. A good death recognizes the inherent dignity of each person and views them as a person to love more than as a problem to solve (or eliminate). Appropriate palliative care and hospice services are utilized and provide meaningful accompaniment.

2. In a good death, meticulous attention is paid to pain and symptom management.

3. In a good death, medications must be selected prudently and judiciously, and pain concerns taken seriously and managed well.

4. A good death looks toward the soul's future with attention to spiritual care. This is a time of profound meaning and continued growth, when spiritual resources and opportunities should be made available.

5. At a good death, a patient should have all their basic needs met (a clean, comfortable, and safe place to be, adequate nutrition and hydration). I believe this is also an essential human right and therefore a larger, societal concern.

6. A good death supports the patient and everyone who loves the patient. The care of a dying patient's loved ones should begin while the patient is still living, with proper grief support and attention to their needs.

7. A good death should be one that is prepared for, as much as possible. Intentional conversations by the patient with their doctors, family members, and friends should be had beforehand regarding the patient's perspective, views, and values with respect to care related to the end of life.

8. A good death should be as natural as possible, not held together by life-sustaining machines. The often-seen contemporary death in the intensive care unit after life-sustaining treatments are withdrawn is not the peaceful, natural ending to life that I hope for.

9. A good death is in God's timing, not one's own. The process happens in its own way; no interventions hasten or cause it.

10. Ultimately, a good death is one where, in the course of the dying process, the patient and their loved ones find meaning, see value, grow, generate positive activity, and share life-affirming interactions. Caring for the dying is not about giving up or facilitating a quick, tidy, and premature death. It is about optimizing human flourishing, love, and even beauty at the end of life.

EPILOGUE

Pope Francis speaks about the "throwaway culture" that says, "'I use you as much as I need you. When I am not interested in you anymore, or you are in my way, I throw you out.' It is especially the weakest who are treated this way—unborn children, the elderly, the needy, and the disadvantaged."[1] Care for the sick and dying must focus on the inherent dignity of the person and the "sacred and unique gift" each human person is: made and loved by God, valuable and precious.

HOW AS CATHOLICS CAN WE ADVOCATE FOR PRO-LIFE, PRO-DIGNITY END-OF-LIFE CARE, AND WARD AGAINST PHYSICIAN-ASSISTED SUICIDE AND EUTHANASIA?

In this section, I am just going to be honest: it is not enough for us Catholics to say that we are opposed to physician-assisted suicide (PAS) and euthanasia. We must take it a step further and advocate for how we believe the sick and dying should be accompanied and respected. This is where I believe pro-life, pro-dignity palliative care to be the true antidote.

I never personally sought out this path I am on, educating others about end-of-life care. Rather, I believe God gave me this mission and did it in a rather dramatic way. The very day after I took my palliative medicine and hospice board exams, the capstone to twelve years of medical education and training, PAS became legal in the state of Colorado, where I had just moved to practice. I wept. I could not believe it. One of the primary reasons I had entered into the subspecialty was to help people with serious illnesses have improved lives: better pain and symptom management, psychosocial support, and richer lives full of meaning not defined by their illness. I was bright-eyed and bushy-tailed, just out of my medical training and enthusiastic to make the world a better place for people stressed by their health situation. I never would have moved somewhere where this was legal! But God knew where I needed to be.

In my opinion, palliative medicine has nothing to do with PAS, but as this law rolled out, it was clear that my opinion was in the minority. Very fortunately, the hospital system for which I worked was able to opt out of involvement with PAS. Never before had I been more grateful to and proud of my employer. But although I was not going to face daily pressure to involve myself with this new law, it did not mean I was exempt from dealing with it. Patients and their family members who did not understand our hospital system's stance would still ask me about PAS and even at times ask me to prescribe the drugs to them. These conversations were always so difficult for me, and I implored the Holy Spirit's assistance to navigate them.

It is tragic how palliative medicine has gotten caught up with this death movement. It has caused tremendous moral distress, as patients have a more difficult time trusting doctors (including myself) because they believe their death is going to be hastened. PAS should not be considered a role of medicine; it is inconsistent with the foundational ethos of the medical profession. I am here to care, not to kill. Once doctors begin killing patients, the trust inherent in the beautiful, sacred, physician-patient relationship is destroyed.

One of the reasons I wrote this book was to increase awareness and understanding about how life, in the midst of today's culture, can be respected in serious illness and at the end of life. In this book I have tried to clarify many of the misunderstandings I have witnessed. For they are not just present in the non-medical laity. In recent years I have witnessed an esteemed priest who wrote an article describing palliative care as "a euphemism for euthanasia." I have encountered well-intentioned Catholic physicians who have discouraged supporting palliative care as a field because it is just too "full of abuses." I have seen diocesan pro-life leaders incorrectly use the terms "palliative care" and "hospice" interchangeably, and do the same for "physician-assisted suicide" and "euthanasia." More than once after a talk, someone has come up to me and asked if because of my line of work I have to go to the Sacrament of Penance all the time, implying that I am often doing immoral things such as hastening the death of patients. (I tell them that I go to Confession regularly because I am taking advantage of the grace of the sacrament in my life, not because of bad things I am doing in my job.) It is clear that confusion regarding end-of-life care leads to mistrust.

I believe the misunderstandings around these issues have created an obstacle that prevents adequate advocacy for the dignity of life around natural death. The misunderstandings undermine the ability to be proactive about education and awareness of difficult issues around serious illness and at the end of life. This is a major problem, because the culture continues to view death and suffering as things to be avoided at all costs, even at the cost of eliminating the sufferer. As physician-assisted suicide laws pass in more states, it is imperative that Catholics understand this issue. I believe it is sadly not a question of *if* physician-assisted suicide will come to more states, but it is a question of *when*. Will you be prepared to help fight this if it comes to your state's legislature or to public vote? We must not simply wait for an issue to arise and then just react and be on the defense. We must properly inform ourselves and others about this issue. It is time to be proactive and on offense.[2] We need to be aware of the state of things and have the formation to recognize the evil while at the same time being aware of a response that is good: pro-dignity palliative care. This must be advocated and championed.

There are many ways to practically get involved with promoting dignity at the end of life. This includes advocating for rights for people with disabilities (as these vulnerable groups are becoming particularly targeted), getting involved with legislative and lobbying work to help testify against this, providing general advocacy and education to your community (whether church, school, neighborhood, friend group, etc., as there are so many misperceptions out there!), and taking what you learned in this book to help witness and champion pro-life, pro-dignity palliative care as a way to respectfully accompany the seriously ill and dying. Debunk erroneous thinking on these issues when you see them. Stay informed on issues related to these topics, particularly around where you live. For yourself and your loved ones, create advance directives in a way that respects life (and share them with your doctors!). And, of course, pray.

HOW CAN I PRAY THROUGH ALL THIS?

Experiencing a serious illness yourself or accompanying a loved one through one is not for the faint of heart. It can feel so overwhelming, and you may feel lost, out of control, and despairing. Your faith life may be put on the back burner as you enter into survival mode, focused on getting through the daily obstacles of this situation. You may feel frustrated, angry, or distant from God and have a sense that he has abandoned you and your family. These are all common.

What I implore and encourage you to do is to not give up on him. I ask you to trust him even in the midst of this great suffering. He is a good God, one who is surely bigger than all this. He knows the deepest parts of our hearts; he knows the number of hairs on our heads. Although why he permitted this to happen is beyond our understanding, we must continue to have faith in him.

Sometimes the best we can muster when we feel so beaten up by life's circumstances is just to show up. To show up to Mass, to show up to Adoration, to show up to prayer. Even if we feel completely dry and that we have nothing to say, nothing to offer, we can keep showing up. I encourage you to be honest with the Lord—he can handle whatever you have to say. And if you need a bit of a start, I have included some prayers that may be helpful. Be assured of my prayers for you. May God bless you and your loved ones.

Prayer in Serious Illness and Suffering
by Natalie King, MD

Dear Lord,
Give me strength to endure this pain.
Give me fortitude to remain mentally strong.
Increase my fidelity to your Church, your promises.
Help me always to recognize the inherent dignity of life,
even at its weakest and most vulnerable.
I give thanks for all who help care for me and ask for your blessing on
    them.
I trust in your goodness, Lord. I believe you can do all things.
If it is your will, please bring an end to this suffering.
Please help me bear this cross
and grant me your peace that goes beyond understanding.

Amen.

Prayer for Those in Chronic Pain

God of Compassion,
you willingly took on our human condition
to experience the same pain, suffering and death that we do.
Through your Son's resurrection,
you transformed suffering and death into new life and glory;
and invite us to join our own pain and struggles to those of Jesus.
Increase the faith and hope of all who are suffering,
especially those living with chronic illness and pain.
Strengthen and confirm in them the promise of new life and glory.
We pray this through the intercession of Our Lady of Lourdes
and in the name of your Son, Jesus
and the Holy Spirit, now and forever.

Amen.[3]

St. Gianna's Prayer

Gianna Beretta Molla was a twentieth-century Italian Roman Catholic pedi-atrician. She is the patron saint of mothers, physicians, and unborn children.

Jesus, I promise to submit myself to all that you permit to befall me,
make me only know your will.
My most sweet Jesus, infinitely merciful God,
most tender Father of souls, and in a particular way of the weak,
most miserable, most infirm which you carry with special tenderness
between your divine arms,
I come to you to ask you, through the love and merits of your Sacred
    Heart,
the grace to comprehend and to do always your holy will,
the grace to confide in you, the grace to rest securely through time and
    eternity in your loving divine arms.

Amen.[4]

Prayer to St. Luke

An apostle and one of the four gospel writers, St. Luke is recognized as the first Christian physician and is the patron saint of physicians and surgeons.

Oh, holy apostle, St. Luke,
I ask your intercession on behalf of all physicians,
particularly those caring for me/my loved ones.
Humbly lay them at the Divine Physician's feet
and ask that they have: the wisdom and knowledge necessary
to treat their patients effectively and restore them to physical and mental
    health;
the compassion and empathy necessary to be of comfort to those who are
    suffering;
and the strength and grace to fulfill their duties as doctors.
I pray that you keep them safe from harm
and that they maintain encouragement despite the challenges before
    them.
O blessed St. Luke, we thank you for your prayers and assistance.

Amen.[5]

Prayer for the Protection of Life at its Natural End
By Natalie King, MD

Dear Lord,

I ask your special protection over all people who are dealing with serious
illness or find themselves nearing the end of their earthly life.

Please fill them with comfort of mind, body, and spirit.

Please give them hope and peace that surpasses all understanding.

Give them strength to endure any trial, any suffering.

Grant them the realization that their life is a gift, and that the God of all
goodness sees them.

Please grant that they are never tempted to consider the premature
hastening of their death.

Lord, I ask you to help people find encouragement during difficult
moments.

Please help protect vulnerable persons and safeguard them from unjust
laws.

I pray that our culture can be one that selflessly loves and cares for the
sick, disabled, and dying to their natural death.

I thank you for your creation and celebrate this beautiful life you gave
me.

Amen.

Prayer to St. Joseph for a Happy Death

O Blessed Joseph, you gave your last breath in the loving embrace of Jesus
and Mary.

When the seal of death shall close my life, come with Jesus and Mary to
aid me.

Obtain for me this solace for that hour—to die with their holy arms
around me.

Jesus, Mary, and Joseph, I commend my soul, living and dying, into your
sacred arms.

Amen.

Prayer of a Catholic Palliative Physician
by Natalie King, MD

Dear Lord,
You know the hearts and hear the pleas
of those who cry out to you for relief in their suffering.
I ask for an increase in strength, in hope,
and in trust of your plan.
And I ask for your mercy.
Confident of your love, help me to best accompany those
who have been put in my path for me to help.
Give me courage to stand up for the vulnerable
and to boldly advocate for the utmost dignity and respect
to be shown toward those nearing the end of their earthly lives.
Please endow me with abundant patience, kindness, and empathy
as I care for others in grief.
May I radiate your love and peace.
When you permit me to experience personal suffering or loss,
help me bear it virtuously.
May I live with confidence in your promise of salvation.

Amen.

ADDITIONAL PRAYER RESOURCES CAN BE FOUND AT:

USCCB Prayers for Death and Dying
https://www.usccb.org/prayers/prayers-death-and-dying

USCCB Prayers for the Health and Dignity of the Sick
https://www.usccb.org/prayers/prayers-health-and-dignity-sick

RELEVANT CHURCH DOCUMENTS AND ADDITIONAL HELPFUL RESOURCES

Following are brief descriptions of what I find are some of the most relevant and helpful resources if you want to learn more about Catholic teaching and tradition as they intersect with healthcare in serious illness and at the end of life.

CATHOLIC HEALTH CARE ETHICS: A MANUAL FOR PRACTITIONERS, 3RD EDITION
Edited by Edward J. Furton, 2020

This is a textbook distributed by the National Catholic Bioethics Center and is an in-depth resource on Catholic bioethical principles and applied issues. It is a practical guide for Catholic healthcare practitioners as well as those who work in Catholic healthcare settings, based in Church documents and providing a bit of a deeper look into many controversial ethical issues.

THE CONVERSATION PROJECT

This is an advance care planning tool to help speak with loved ones about care values and preferences. I particularly like the "Conversation Starter Guide." https://theconversationproject.org

ETHICAL AND RELIGIOUS DIRECTIVES FOR CATHOLIC HEALTH CARE SERVICES, 6TH EDITION
United States Conference of Catholic Bishops, 2018

This document is a series of directives from the bishops' conference that provides moral guidance in applying Catholic ethical principles to health-care delivery. Catholic hospitals and healthcare systems, as part of their Catholic identity, follow these. www.usccb.org/resources/ethical-and-religious-directives-catholic-healthcare-services

EVANGELIUM VITAE ("THE GOSPEL OF LIFE," ON THE VALUE AND INVIOLABILITY OF HUMAN LIFE)
Encyclical by Pope St. John Paul II, 1995

In this encyclical, Pope St. John Paul II emphasizes the inherent dignity of life and its sacred inviolability. He sheds light on the threats to human life becoming ever more prevalent in today's culture, particularly at the beginning and end of life with abortion and euthanasia. www.vatican.va/content/john-paul-ii/en/encyclicals/documents/hf_jp-ii_enc_25031995_evangelium-vitae.html

The USCCB's website has a two-page summary. www.usccb.org/resources/wwmin-evangelium-vitae-summary.pdf

GET PALLIATIVE CARE
This is a resource with general information about palliative care. I particularly like the handout for patients and families and have often handed it out during consultations if patients are unfamiliar with what I do or why I may have been asked to see them. https://getpalliativecare.org

NATIONAL CATHOLIC BIOETHICS CENTER (NCBC)
The NCBC is a nonprofit research organization led by Catholic ethicists that provides education and appropriate application of Church teachings to complex medical situations. They have many helpful publications, links to a variety of ethics-related Church documents on their website, and a

24/7 Catholic bioethicist support line that is available to support health-care professionals and laity. www.NCBCenter.org

NOW AND AT THE HOUR OF OUR DEATH: CATHOLIC GUIDANCE FOR END-OF-LIFE DECISION MAKING

This website resource from the New York State Catholic Conference has an overview of Catholic end-of-life teaching and links to Catholic and state-specific advance directive information. www.catholicendoflife.org

RESPONSES TO CERTAIN QUESTIONS OF THE UNITED STATES CONFERENCE OF CATHOLIC BISHOPS CONCERNING ARTIFICIAL NUTRITION AND HYDRATION, WITH COMMENTARY

Dicastery for the Doctrine of the Faith, 2007

This offers a deeper look at the Church's view on artificial nutrition and hydration. www.vatican.va/roman_curia/congregations/cfaith/documents/ rc_con_cfaith_doc_20070801_risposte-usa_en.html

SALVIFICI DOLORIS ("SALVIFIC SUFFERING," ON THE CHRISTIAN MEANING OF HUMAN SUFFERING)

Apostolic Letter by Pope St. John Paul II, 1984

In this letter, Pope St. John Paul II delves into the spiritual significance of suffering and its redemptive value. He helps us understand how to get meaning out of suffering and how to practically best live out our own suffering.   www.vatican.va/content/john-paul-ii/en/apost_letters/1984/ documents/hf_jp-ii_apl_11021984_salvifici-doloris.html

SAMARITANUS BONUS ("THE GOOD SAMARITAN," ON THE CARE OF PERSONS IN THE CRITICAL AND TERMINAL PHASES OF LIFE)

Dicastery for the Doctrine of the Faith, 2020

In this document, the Dicastery for the Doctrine of the Faith provides the Catholic response to many issues surrounding serious illness and death in today's culture. It sheds light on the concept of accompaniment of the suffering other, following the example of the Good Samaritan. It also asserts the good of palliative care. It is a helpful document for all who come into contact with the sick and dying: physicians, nurses, other healthcare workers, family members, priests, and other pastoral workers. www.vatican. va/roman_curia/congregations/cfaith/documents/rc_con_cfaith_ doc_20200714_samaritanus-bonus_en.html

NOTES

1. MEDICAL CARE IN SERIOUS ILLNESS AND AT THE END OF LIFE

1. Source: Paige Comstock Barker and Jennifer S. Scherer, "Illness Trajectories: Description and Clinical Use," Palliative Care Network of Wisconsin, March 6, 2019, https://www.mypcnow.org/fast-fact/illness-trajectories-description-and-clinical-use/.

2. See, for example, Jarred Cinman, "The Five Best Reasons Not to Believe in God," Daily Maverick, February 26, 2015, https://www.dailymaverick.co.za/opinionista/2015-02-26-the-five-best-reasons-not-to-believe-in-god/.

2. PALLIATIVE MEDICINE AND HOSPICE 101

1. The pallium is a liturgical vestment worn by popes, archbishops, and bishops. It is bestowed by a pope on archbishops and bishops to symbolize their participation in papal authority over a particular jurisdiction. It is made of a circular strip of white lamb's wool and placed over the shoulders.

2. "About Palliative Care," Center to Advance Palliative Care, https://www.capc.org/about/palliative-care/. The Center to Advance Palliative Care (CAPC) is a helpful resource for both patients and healthcare workers.

3. Jennifer S. Temel et al., "Early Palliative Care for Patients with Metastatic Non-Small-Cell-Lung Cancer," *New England Journal of Medicine* 363, no. 8 (August 19, 2010): 733–42, https://www.nejm.org/doi/full/10.1056/nejmoa1000678.

4. Temel et al., "Early Palliative Care."

5. See Henry Brodaty, "Family Caregivers of People with Dementia," *Dialogues in Clinical Neuroscience* 11, no. 2 (June 2009): 217–28, https://www.ncbi.nlm.nih.gov/pmc/articles/PMC3181916/.

3. COMMUNICATION AROUND SERIOUS ILLNESS

1. Questions adapted from Johanna Turner, "Conversations with Your Physician about Serious Illness: Being Heard, Getting Answers," American Hospice Foundation, https://americanhospice.org/learning-about-hospice/conversations-with-your-physician-about-serious-illness-being-heard-getting-answers/.

4. NAVIGATING TREATMENT OPTIONS

1. United States Conference of Catholic Bishops, *Ethical and Religious Directives for Catholic Health Care Services*, 6th ed. (Washington, DC: USCCB, 2018), https://www.usccb.org/resources/ethical-religious-direc-tives-catholic-health-service-sixth-edition-2016-06_0.pdf.
2. See *Samaritanus Bonus*, sec. 5, no. 7, for further details.

5. ADVANCE CARE PLANNING

1. Paul S. Applebaum, "Assessment of Patients' Competence to Consent to Treatment," *New England Journal of Medicine* 357, no. 18 (2007): 1834–40.
2. Peter Morrow, "The Catholic Living Will and Healthcare Surrogate: A Teaching Document for Evangelization and a Means of Ensuring Spirituality throughout Life," *Linacre Quarterly* 80, no. 4 (November 2013): 317–22.

6. UNDERSTANDING THE DYING PROCESS

1. Content from this chapter was adapted from Nathan E. Goldstein and R. Sean Morrison, *Evidence-Based Practice of Palliative Medicine* (Philadelphia: Saunders, 2012).
2. Peter A. Singer, Douglas K. Martin, and Merrijoy Kelner, "Quality End-of-Life Care: Patients' Perspectives," *JAMA* 281, no. 2 (1999): 163–68, doi:10.1001/jama.281.2.163.

3. Pope John Paul II, "Address to the Participants in the International Congress on 'Life-Sustaining Treatments and Vegetative State: Scientific Advances and Ethical Dilemmas'" (March 20, 2004), no. 4 (emphasis in original), https://www.vatican.va/content/john-paul-ii/en/speeches/2004/march/documents/hf_jp-ii_spe_20040320_congress-fiamc.html.

4. Ira Byock, *Dying Well: Peace and Possibilities at the End of Life* (New York: Riverhead Books, 1998).

7. PREMATURE HASTENING OF DEATH

1. "Fourth Annual Report on Medical Assistance in Dying in Canada 2022," Canada.ca, October 2023, https://www.canada.ca/en/health-canada/services/publications/health-system-services/annual-report-medical-assistance-dying-2022.html#chart_3.1.

2. To learn more about Catholic teaching on suicide, see *Responding to Suicide: A Pastoral Handbook for Catholic Leaders*, compiled and edited by Deacon Ed Shoener and Bishop John Dolan (Notre Dame, IN: Ave Maria Press, 2020).

3. Timothy E. Quill and Franklin G. Miller, ed., *Palliative Care and Ethics* (New York: Oxford University Press, 2014), 155.

4. Pope John Paul II, "Address to the Participants in the 19th International Conference of the Pontifical Council for Health Pastoral Care" (November 12, 2004), https://www.vatican.va/content/john-paul-ii/en/speeches/2004/november/documents/hf_jp-ii_spe_20041112_pc-hlth-work.html

5. Pope Benedict XVI, "Message for the Fifteenth World Day of the Sick" (December 8, 2006), https://www.vatican.va/content/benedict-xvi/en/messages/sick/documents/hf_ben-xvi_mes_20061208_world-day-of-the-sick-2007.html.

6. Pope Francis, "Address to Participants in the Plenary of the Pontifical Academy for Life" (March 5, 2015), https://www.vatican.va/content/francesco/en/speeches/2015/march/documents/papa-francesco_20150305_pontificia-accademia-vita.html.

7. "Statement on Physician-Assisted Dying," American Academy of Hospice and Palliative Medicine, June 24, 2016, https://aahpm.org/positions/pad.

9. PARTICULARLY DIFFICULT TOPICS

1. Marie T. Nolan, "Ethical Issues in Organ Donation and Transplantation," in *Catholic Health Care Ethics: A Manual for Practitioners*, 3rd ed., ed. Edward J. Furton (Philadelphia: National Catholic Bioethics Center, 2020).

2. R. R. Nash and C. E. Thiele, "Informing Consent for Organ Donation," *HEC Forum* 28, no. 3 (2016): 187–91, doi:10.1007/s10730-016-9304-1.

3. G. T. Brown, "Medical Futility in Concept, Culture, and Practice," *Journal of Clinical Ethics* 29, no. 1 (2018): 114–23, PMID: 30129737.

10. PORTRAIT OF A PALLIATIVE MEDICINE PHYSICIAN

1. Jeffrey P. Bishop, *The Anticipatory Corpse: Medicine, Power, and the Care of the Dying* (Notre Dame, IN: University of Notre Dame Press, 2011), 3.

EPILOGUE

1. Quoted in Courtney Mares, "Pope Francis Decries Culture That 'Throws Away' Unborn Children, Elderly, Poor," Catholic News Agency, January 29, 2023, https://www.catholicnewsagency.com/news/253492/pope-francis-decries-culture-that-throws-away-unborn-children-elderly-poor.

2. See Charles C. Camosy, "A Glimpse into a Post-Christian Future: Public Support for Killing the Poor and Disabled," Public Discourse, June 12, 2023, https://www.thepublicdiscourse.com/2023/06/89216/.

3. Catholic Health Association of the United States, https://www.chausa.org/prayers/additional-resources/2018-month-of-prayer/prayer-for-those-in-chronic-pain.

4. St. Gianna's Center for Women's Health and Fertility Care, https://www.stgiannacenter.com/st-giannas-prayer/.

5. Adapted from Ann Fitch, "Prayer to St. Luke," Practical Prayers, https://practicalprayers.com/prayer-saint-luke-doctors/.

Natalie King, MD, is a palliative medicine physician who cares for patients with serious illness and those nearing the end of life. King writes and speaks nationally, educating about and advocating for the expansion of palliative medicine as the surest way to safeguard human dignity in serious illness and end-of-life care.

After finishing her medical training, King worked as a palliative medicine physician for several years at a hospital in Colorado, where she led the hospital's ethics committee and helped teach trainees. She partnered with the USCCB to improve education for Catholic laity about palliative care and organized a forum for the Catholic Medical Association on end-of-life issues.

King holds a bachelor of arts degree in anthropology and pre-professional studies from the University of Notre Dame, a master of arts degree in bioethics from the Ohio State University College of Medicine, and a doctor of medicine degree from Tulane University School of Medicine.

She lives with her family in Utah.

nataliekingmd.com